Radiation Medicine Rounds

Charles R. Thomas, Jr., MD

Editor-in-Chief

Professor and Chair
Department of Radiation Medicine
Professor, Division of Hematology/Oncology
Department of Medicine
Knight Cancer Institute
Oregon Health & Science University Cancer Institute
Portland, Oregon

Editorial Board

Forthcoming Issues

Radiation Medicine Rounds

VOLUME 2, ISSUE 3

Gynecologic Cancer

Guest Editors

Arno J. Mundt, MD
Catheryn M. Yashar, MD
Loren K. Mell, MD
Department of Radiation Oncology
University of California San Diego
San Diego, California

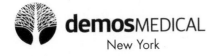

demosMEDICAL
New York

Acquisitions Editor: Richard Winters
Cover Design: Joe Tenerelli
Compositor: Newgen Imaging
Printer: Bradford & Bigelow

Visit our website at www.demosmedpub.com

Radiation Medicine Rounds is published three times a year by Demos Medical Publishing.

Business Office. All business correspondence including subscriptions, renewals, and address changes should be sent to Demos Medical Publishing, 11 West 42nd Street, 15th Floor, New York, NY, 10036.

ISSN: 2151-4208
ISBN: 978-1-936287-47-5
E-ISBN: 978-1-617050-95-4

Library of Congress Cataloging-in-Publication Data

Gynecologic cancer / guest editors, Arno J. Mundt, Catheryn M. Yashar, Loren K. Mell.
   p. ; cm. -- (Radiation medicine rounds, ISSN 2151-4208 ; v. 2, issue 3)
  Includes bibliographical references and index.
  ISBN 978-1-936287-47-5 (alk. paper) -- ISBN 978-1-61705-095-4 (e-ISBN)
  I. Mundt, Arno J. II. Yashar, Catheryn M. III. Mell, Loren K. IV. Series: Radiation medicine rounds ; v. 2, Issue 3. 2151-4208
  [DNLM: 1. Genital Neoplasms, Female--therapy. W1 RA162HD v.2 issue 3 / WP 145]

  616.99'46506--dc23

             2011043804

Reprints. For copies of 100 or more of articles in this publication, please contact Reina Santana, Special Sales Manager.

Special discounts on bulk quantities of Demos Medical Publishing books are available to corporations, professional associations, pharmaceutical companies, health care organizations, and other qualifying groups. For details, please contact:

Reina Santana, Special Sales Manager
Demos Medical Publishing LLC
11 W. 42nd Street
New York, NY 10036
Phone: 800-532-8663 or 212-683-0072
Fax: 212-941-7842
E-mail: rsantana@demosmedpub.com

Made in the United States of America
11 12 13   14   15   5 4 3 2 1

Contents

Foreword

■ FROM THE EDITOR-IN-CHIEF

Radiation Medicine Rounds is a hardcover periodical published three times a year that is designed to provide an up-to-date review of dedicated radiation medicine topics of interest to clinicians and scientists who are involved in the care of patients receiving radiotherapy. It is intended to serve as both a reference and an instructional tool by students, housestaff, fellows, practicing clinicians, medical physicists, cancer biologists, radiobiologists, and interdisciplinary colleagues throughout the oncology spectrum.

For the current issue, *Gynecologic Cancer*, Guest Editors Drs. Arno J. Mundt, Catheryn M. Yashar, and Loren K. Mell have assembled a cast of highly respected thought leaders in the art of gynecologic radiation oncology. They are to be praised for delivering a well-researched, timely, and user-friendly product that covers the state of the art for tumors of the female abdominal and pelvic reproductive tract. On behalf of the entire *Radiation Medicine Rounds* editorial board, I congratulate Drs. Mundt, Yashar, and Mell for putting together an outstanding contribution that will be useful to colleagues who are involved in the delivery of clinical care to patients requiring radiotherapy for the major gynecologic solid tumors.

Dr. Charles R. Thomas, Jr.
Series Editor-in-Chief
Radiation Medicine Rounds
Portland, Oregon

Preface

The management of patients with gynecologic cancers is truly multidisciplinary, requiring close interaction and collaboration between gynecologic oncologists, medical oncologists, and radiation oncologists. This is becoming increasingly true today as novel procedures and treatments are being developed in all three fields. We thus felt it was essential to seek out leading clinicians and researchers in these disciplines, highlighting current cutting-edge approaches for this volume of *Radiation Medicine Rounds*.

The initial section is devoted to novel radiation approaches, including intensity-modulated radiation therapy and image-guided radiation therapy, in the planning and treatment of both external beam irradiation and brachytherapy. The subsequent section focuses on the role of chemotherapy and novel biologic agents in the treatment of gynecologic cancers. Surgical approaches are highlighted next, including the current role of lymphadenectomy in endometrial cancer and the emerging role of robotic-assisted surgery in gynecologic cancers in general. Finally, an overview of the use of magnetic resonance imaging as a means of assessing tumor response in cervical cancer patients undergoing treatment is presented.

It is our sincere hope that this *Gynecologic Cancer* volume succeeds in portraying the multidisciplinary nature of gynecologic cancer management and will serve as a helpful and instructive reference for both clinicians and researchers alike.

Arno J. Mundt, MD
Catheryn M. Yashar, MD
Loren K. Mell, MD

Contributors

Sushil Beriwal, MD
Department of Radiation Oncology
University of Pittsburgh Cancer Institute
Pittsburgh, PA

David A. Clump, MD, PhD
Department of Radiation Oncology
University of Pittsburgh Cancer Institute
Pittsburgh, PA

Madeleine Courtney-Brooks, MD, MPH
Department of Obstetrics and Gynecology
University of Virginia
Charlottesville, VA

Linda R. Duska, MD
Department of Obstetrics and Gynecology
University of Virginia
Charlottesville, VA

Marilyn Huang, MD, MS
Department of Gynecologic Oncology &
    Reproductive Medicine
MD Anderson Cancer Center
Houston, TX

Zhibin Huang, PhD
Department of Radiation Oncology
East Carolina University
Greenville, NC

Lindsay G. Jensen, MAS
Department of Radiation Oncology
University of California San Diego
La Jolla, CA

Mitch Kamrava, MD
Department of Radiation Oncology
University of California Los Angeles
Los Angeles, CA

Simon S. Lo, MD
Department of Radiation Oncology
Case Western Reserve University
Cleveland, OH

Vicky Makker, MD
Gynecologic Medical Oncology Service
Memorial Sloan Kettering Cancer
    Center
New York, NY

Nina A. Mayr, MD
Department of Radiation Oncology
Ohio State University
Columbus, OH

Donald Scott McMeekin, MD
Department of Obstetrics and
    Gynecology
University of Oklahoma Health Science
    Center
Oklahoma, OK

Loren K. Mell, MD
Department of Radiation Oncology
University of California San Diego
La Jolla, CA

Arno J. Mundt, MD
Department of Radiation Oncology
University of California San Diego
La Jolla, CA

Elizabeth Kathleen Nugent, MD
Department of Obstetrics and Gynecology
University of Oklahoma Health Science
    Center
Oklahoma, OK

Pedro Ramirez, MD
Department of Gynecologic Oncology &
    Reproductive Medicine
MD Anderson Cancer Center
Houston, TX

Akila N. Viswanathan, MD, MPH
Department of Radiation Oncology
Brigham and Women's Hospital/
    Dana-Farber Cancer Institute
Harvard Medical School
Boston, MA

Catheryn M. Yashar, MD
Department of Radiation Oncology
University of California San Diego
La Jolla, CA

William T. C. Yuh, MD, MSEE
Department of Radiology
Ohio State University
Columbus, OH

Radiation Medicine Rounds

VOLUME 2, ISSUE 3

Gynecologic Cancer

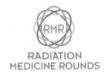

RADIATION
MEDICINE ROUNDS

Intensity-Modulated Radiotherapy for Gynecologic Malignancies

Lindsay G. Jensen, Arno J. Mundt, and Loren K. Mell*

Department of Radiation Oncology, University of California San Diego, La Jolla, CA

■ ABSTRACT

The use of intensity-modulated radiotherapy (IMRT) for gynecologic malignancies has increased significantly over the last decade. IMRT planning techniques and normal tissue dose constraints are becoming well-established, particularly for cervical and endometrial cancers. Dosimetric studies comparing IMRT and conventional techniques have been conducted for most gynecologic cancers, in general showing that IMRT provides equal or increased target dose while sparing dose to surrounding normal tissues. Initial outcome studies have reported decreased toxicity and comparable disease control with IMRT compared with conventional radiotherapy (RT). Novel applications such as bone-marrow-sparing IMRT, simultaneous integrated boost, and hypofractionated stereotactic body RT (SBRT) provide treatment alternatives that are difficult to obtain using conventional techniques. Prospective multi-institutional clinical trials with long-term follow-up are still needed to establish the effects of IMRT on disease control, toxicity, and quality of life.

Keywords: IMRT, gynecologic cancer, pelvic organ motion

■ INTRODUCTION

Conventional radiotherapy (RT) techniques for gynecologic malignancies typically involve opposed anterior/posterior–posterior/anterior, with or without opposed lateral fields, to treat the primary site or postoperative bed and regional lymph nodes. Frequently, bone landmarks are used to design radiation ports, without explicit target or normal tissue delineation. Conventional RT is associated with multiple acute and late adverse effects, including diarrhea, malabsorption, myelosuppression, pelvic fractures, bowel obstructions, perforations, or fistulae (1,2). These complications have a significant adverse impact on quality of life and can limit patients' tolerance to intensive treatment (3).

Intensity-modulated radiotherapy (IMRT) is a technique that can reduce dose to surrounding organs at risk (OARs) while maintaining high target doses. IMRT holds considerable promise to reduce radiation-associated complications and increase the therapeutic ratio of RT. The use of IMRT for gynecologic malignancies has increased significantly over the last decade (4), but prospective studies supporting its use are limited, and randomized trials establishing its benefits compared to conventional

---

*Corresponding author, Department of Radiation Oncology, 3855 Health Sciences Drive, MC0843, La Jolla, CA 92093

E-mail address: lmell@ucsd.edu

Radiation Medicine Rounds 2:3 (2011) 341–356.
DOI: 10.5003/2151–4208.2.3.341

techniques are lacking. This review will discuss techniques, dosimetric advantages, planning techniques, clinical outcomes studies, challenges, and future directions in the use of IMRT to treat gynecologic malignancies.

■ PELVIC RT

Dosimetric Studies

Multiple dosimetric studies have found that IMRT achieves similar target coverage and decreases dose to pelvic organs compared to conventional planning for pelvic RT (5–12). An initial study by Roeske et al. (5) found that in women with cervical and endometrial cancer, IMRT reduced the proportion of bladder, rectum, and small bowel irradiated at the prescription dose by 23, 23, and 50%, respectively, compared with conventional four-field box plans. Similarly, Heron et al. (6) found that IMRT reduced the volume of bladder, rectum, and small bowel receiving >30 Gy by 36, 66, and 52%, respectively, compared with conventional techniques. Guo et al. (7) also compared three-dimensional conformal RT (3DCRT) with IMRT for 10 endometrial cancer patients and found that IMRT reduced the fraction of small bowel, rectum, and bladder receiving >45 Gy by 18, 26, and 43%, respectively.

Studies have also found dosimetric advantages of alternative intensity-modulated pelvic RT techniques. For example, Yang et al. (8) found that helical tomotherapy decreased dose to bladder and rectum and improved homogeneity compared with conventional techniques, but this technique also increased integral dose to bowel and pelvic bones. Cozzi et al. (9) compared intensity-modulated arc therapy (IMAT) with IMRT plans for eight cervical cancer patients and found that IMAT increased homogeneity and conformity and decreased dose to rectum, bladder, and small bowel. Wong et al. (10) also found that IMAT decreased dose to small bowel and iliac bone marrow, while maintaining adequate planning target volume (PTV) dose. IMAT also offers an advantage over IMRT of shorter beam-on time. Using a pseudo step-wedge intensity-modulated (PSWIM) technique, Macdonald et al. (11) showed that significantly higher dose could be delivered to point A and point P, with similar rectal doses. Bladder point dose was higher with PSWIM than with standard

IMRT or conventional RT; of 10 patients treated with this techniques, none experienced grade >2 acute toxicity.

Although IMRT has been studied primarily in cervical and endometrial cancer, planning studies in other gynecologic sites have shown similar advantages. For example, Cilla et al. (12) evaluated IMRT plans compared with 3DCRT plans for postoperative vaginal cancer patients and found that IMRT improved conformity and decreased rectal and bladder doses.

Treatment Planning and Delivery

Computed tomography (CT) simulation is used for IMRT planning. Many, if not most, IMRT users simulate patients in the supine position (13). However, prone IMRT may further decrease bowel dose compared with supine IMRT. Adli et al. (14) compared prone and supine positioning for limited and extended arc techniques and found decreased dose to small bowel with prone positioning, but variable effects for large bowel dose. Another planning study (15) indicated that prone position had similar target coverage to supine position with decreased the volume of small bowel irradiated to ≥20 Gy (V_{20}), but increased the volume of rectum irradiated between 10 and 40 Gy. Huh et al. (16) found that combining prone positioning with a customized small bowel displacement system decreased small bowel dose at all levels from 5 to 105% of the prescription dose. It is uncertain, however, if the dosimetric advantages of prone positioning translate into decreased toxicity. For example, Beriwal et al. (17) compared 47 consecutive patients treated in the prone and supine position and did not find significant differences in dose to bowel or in rates of toxicity between the two groups.

Oral and intravenous contrast agents are generally recommended to aid target delineation. Immobilization is important due to the steeper dose gradients with IMRT, as inaccurate setup could decrease target dose and increase normal tissue dose. Custom immobilization devices, such as an alpha cradle, are recommended and can reduce setup errors to <5 mm (18). While CT is used most commonly for treatment planning in cervical cancer patients (19), magnetic resonance imaging (MRI) may show important soft tissue differences that cannot be seen on CT. MRI appears to be more accurate than CT in assessing uterine invasion and delineating tumor volumes (20), but use of MRI can be limited by cost and availability. ^{18}F-fluorodeoxyglucose (^{18}F-FDG)-positron emission tomography (PET) has a high specificity for diseased lymph nodes (21) and is therefore useful in treatment planning for defining a nodal boost volume. Fusion of MRI and/or PET to the planning CT, when available, is generally recommended to augment targeting. Novel imaging techniques such as (60)-Cu-ATSM PET, which is used to identify hypoxic cells, have also been implemented in cervical cancer treatment planning (22), but such technologies are not in widespread use.

Consensus guidelines now exist for the delineation of clinical target volume (CTV) for postoperative cervical and endometrial cancer (Figure 1) (23) as well as intact cervical cancer (Figure 2) (24), but have not yet been established for other gynecological sites. The CTV for intact cervical cancer includes the entire gross tumor volume (GTV), uterus, cervix, and parametria. The upper one-half, two-thirds, or the entire vagina are included in patients with no vaginal involvement, upper vaginal involvement, and extensive vaginal involvement, respectively. The nodal CTV includes the common, internal and external iliac nodes as well as the presacral nodes in cervical cancer patients and in endometrial cancer patients with parametrial involvement. Because lymph nodes are not directly visible on CT, they are included in the CTV by contouring 7 mm around the iliac

vessels. An atlas has been proposed to guide in contouring for postoperative pelvic IMRT (25) and instructional contouring videos have been made available for a multicenter clinical trial of IMRT (26). Several studies have sought to address the size of planning margins required for IMRT planning (27–33). These are discussed later in this review in the section Inter- and Intrafraction Motion.

Normal tissue complication probability (NTCP) analysis has been used to define optimal normal tissue and target input parameters and guidelines for IMRT plan evaluation. For example, Roeske et al. (34) found that the volume of bowel receiving ≥45 Gy (V_{45}) was the most significant risk factor for acute gastrointestinal (GI) toxicity in a cohort of 50 women treated for gynecologic malignancies. Similarly, Simpson et al. (35), in a study of 50 cervical cancer patients undergoing concurrent chemoradiotherapy, found that an increase in the bowel V_{45} of 100 cc was associated with a 2-fold increase in the odds of Radiation Therapy Oncology Group (RTOG) grade ≥2 GI toxicity. Quantitative Analysis of Normal Tissue Effects in the Clinic (QUANTEC) issued recommendations in 2010 (36) to maintain bowel $V_{15} < 120$ cc if individual bowel loops are outlined or $V_{45} < 195$ cc if the entire peritoneal potential space of bowel is outlined. NTCP analysis has been used similarly for defining planning constraints for bone-marrow-sparing IMRT, which is discussed later in this review.

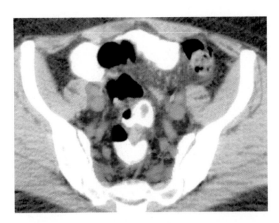

FIGURE 1 Mid-pelvic CT image illustrating a CTV delineated in a patient with cervical cancer treated postoperatively based on guidelines developed for the RTOG 0418 trial. Upper external and internal iliac (red) and presacral region (blue).
Source: Printed with permission from Ref. (23).

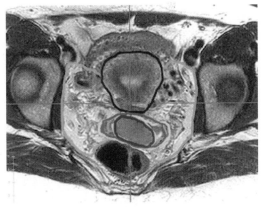

FIGURE 2 Axial view of a T2-weighted MRI illustrating contours of the GTV (red), cervix (pink), vagina (yellow), parametria (green), and uterus (blue) in a patient with intact cervical cancer undergoing IMRT based on the RTOG consensus conference.
Source: Printed with permission from Ref. (24).

Active protocols involving IMRT include the RTOG 0724 trial, a phase III trial of adjuvant carboplatin/paclitaxel in postoperative cervical cancer, and the International Evaluation of Radiotherapy Technology Effectiveness in Cervical Cancer (INTERTECC), a phase II/III trial testing IMRT versus four-field box RT for both postoperative and intact cervix cancer. For the RTOG 0724 trial, either IMRT or conventional RT can be used. An internal target volume (ITV), which is discussed later in this review, is required for IMRT planning on the RTOG 0724 trial, and is optional (but encouraged particularly if daily image guidance is not used) on the INTERTECC trial. Both trials use 45 or 50.4 Gy in 1.8 Gy daily fractions. A comparison of dose-volume guidelines for target and normal tissue structures for the two trials is given in the Table 1.

Toxicity and Outcomes

Postoperative Cervical and Endometrial Cancer

Initial studies of IMRT for cervical and endometrial cancer found that IMRT was associated with decreased rates of acute and chronic toxicity (37–39) compared with four-field box techniques. Mundt et al. (38) found that in a series of 40 endometrial and cervical cancer patients treated with IMRT (70% postoperative), none experience grade ≥3 acute GI toxicity. The percent of women needing no or infrequent antidiarrheal medications during treatment was 75% in the IMRT group compared with 34% with conventional RT. These investigators separately reported on 31 patients treated with IMRT for endometrial cancer; no pelvic failures were observed at 2 years (40).

Beriwal et al. (41) also reported no pelvic, paraaortic, or vaginal recurrences in a group of 47 endometrial cancer patients treated with IMRT. Tierney et al. (42) similarly observed no acute grade ≥3 GI or genitourinary (GU) toxicity; however, 64% of the patients undergoing chemotherapy had grade ≥3 hematologic toxicity. Bouchard et al. (43) reported a series of 15 endometrial cancer patients treated with aperture-based IMRT (AB-IMRT); none had any evidence of recurrence at 27-month follow-up, compared with five recurrences in 30 patients treated with conventional RT. They found that AB-IMRT

TABLE 1 Comparison of dosimetric constraints on active multi-center trials involving IMRT

	RTOG 0724	**INTERTECC**	
PTV	Prescription isodose covers 97% of the PTV	99% prescription isodose encompasses ≥90% of the PTV	
	Volume <93% of prescription dose <0.03 cc	≥99% of the PTV receives ≥90% of the prescription dose	
		≥97% of the PTV receives ≥97% of the prescription dose	
	Volume >110% of prescription dose <0.03 cc	<1% of the PTV receives ≥115% of the prescription dose	
		<10% of the PTV receives ≥110% of the prescription dose	
		Dose max occurs within the PTV	
OARs		*Soft Constraint*	*Hard Constraint*
Bowel	30% receiving ≤40 Gy	V_{45} < 200 cc; max < 50 Gy	V_{45} < 250 cc; max < 110%
Rectum	60% receiving ≤40 Gy	V_{45} < 50%; V_{30} < 60%; max < 50 Gy	Max < 110%
Bladder	35% receiving ≤45 Gy	V_{45} < 50%; max < 50 Gy	Max < 110%
Kidneys	2/3 of each ≤18 Gy	NS	NS
Spinal Cord	Max dose ≤45 Gy	NS	NS
Bone Marrow	NS	V_{10} < 80%; V_{20} < 66%	V_{10} < 90%; V_{20} < 75%
Femoral Head	NS	V_{30} < 15%; max < 50 Gy	Max < 110%

NS: not specified; soft constraints are planning goals, hard constraints are guidelines for plan evaluation.

reduced the volumes of bowel and bladder receiving high dose compared to four-field plans, but did not observe a significant decrease in toxicity compared with historical controls treated conventionally.

Chen et al. (44) studied 68 women treated with postoperative RT (35 conventional, 33 IMRT) and brachytherapy. They found lower rates of acute and chronic GI and GU toxicity in the IMRT group, with similar locoregional control. For 22 postoperative patients included in the study by Hasselle et al. (45), the IMRT group had 100 and 95% 3-year overall and disease-free survival, respectively, with only one patient experiencing grade ≥3 acute toxicity. RTOG 0418, a phase II study to evaluate toxicity and outcomes for IMRT in women with postoperative endometrial and cervical cancer, accrued 106 patients (58 endometrial, 48 cervical). Preliminary results have been reported in abstract form, with 11 of 42 (28%) evaluable endometrial cancer patients and 9 of 40 (23%) cervical cancer patients developing grade ≥2 acute GI toxicity (46,47).

Schwarz et al. (48) recently reported results of a phase I/II trial of helical tomotherapy for postoperative cervical cancer. Twenty-four women were enrolled, with 18 receiving chemotherapy. Median follow-up was 24 months. Grade 3 GI toxicity was observed in 50% of patients, and grade ≥3 hematologic toxicity was 84%. Two late toxicities occurred (vesicovaginal fistula at 25 months and small bowel obstruction at 30 months). The overall and progression-free survival rates at 3 years for all patients were 100 and 89%, respectively.

Intact Cervical Cancer

Several large retrospective series have recently reported outcomes for IMRT in the treatment of intact cervical cancer (45,49,50). Kidd et al. (49) compared 135 IMRT patients with 317 non-IMRT historical controls and found significantly lower rates of grade ≥3 bladder and bowel toxicity in patients treated with IMRT (6%) compared with those treated with whole pelvic RT (17%). They found no difference in posttreatment PET scans between the IMRT and non-IMRT groups and also found improved cause specific and overall survival in the IMRT patients ($p < .0001$).

Hasselle et al. (45) studied 111 cervical cancer patients (89 intact, 22 postoperative) and found 3-year overall survival and disease-free survival of 78 and 69%, respectively. Chen et al. (50) reported

a series of 109 women with 32.5 months median follow-up. The 3-year overall and disease-free survival were similar (78 and 68%, respectively). In both studies, acute grade ≥3 GI toxicity was very low (2–3%). Because acute toxicity has been reported to lead to treatment breaks and missed cycles of chemotherapy, which in turn are predictors of worse overall survival and disease-free survival (51,52), these findings indicate that IMRT has the potential to improve overall treatment delivery and disease outcomes by improving treatment delivery.

Studies in women with cervical cancer treated with helical tomotherapy are limited. Hsieh et al. (53) found 67 and 77% overall and disease-free survival at 2 years, respectively, in a group of 10 women treated with helical tomotherapy. Grade 3 GI toxicity, thrombocytopenia, and leukopenia were observed in 1 (10%), 1 (10%), and 3 (30%) patients, respectively.

Vaginal Cancer

Vera et al. (54) reported on 13 patients treated with IMRT at MD Anderson, with a median follow-up of 18 months. There were no pelvic recurrences observed, and the projected 3-year survival was 75%. Two patients developed fistulas at 3 and 5 months posttreatment.

■ EXTENDED-FIELD RT

Dosimetric Studies

IMRT may allow for dose escalation in high-risk gynecological cancer patients, such as those with paraaortic nodal involvement. Extended-field (EFRT) with concurrent cisplatin is the treatment of choice for this population, but dose escalation and systemic treatment are limited by high rates of acute and chronic toxicity. Several dosimetric studies have shown that extended-field IMRT (EF-IMRT) can decrease the dose to normal tissues including the bladder, rectum, bowel, bone marrow, and kidneys in cervical cancer patients (55–57). For example, Portelance et al. (57) found that the bowel V_{45} could be reduced more than 2-fold with IMRT compared with two- and four-field conventional techniques.

Lian et al. (58) compared IMRT, helical tomotherapy, and 3DCRT for extended-field treatment in stage IIIC endometrial cancer patients and found more conformal PTV coverage using helical tomotherapy and IMRT. Investigators at Washington

University have evaluated the use of PET guided EF-IMRT to escalate dose to paraaortic nodes, primary tumor and involved lymph nodes to 50.4, 59.4, and 59.4 Gy, respectively, for cervical carcinoma (59,60). On average, 97.6% and 89% of the primary tumor/involved lymph nodes and paraaortic nodes received 100% of prescription dose while maintaining the dose to surrounding organs at acceptable levels. They have also published protocol guidelines and are evaluating this technique in prospective clinical trial (60).

Treatment Planning and Delivery

EFRT is delivered in the supine position with treatment fields identical to those used for cervical or endometrial cancer, with the superior border of the field extended up to as high as the T12-L1 intervertebral space, depending on the highest level of lymph node involvement. Normal tissue planning constraints are not well-established for EF-IMRT and vary between studies. Lian et al. (58) used the following planning constraints: bladder (maximal dose, 50 Gy; <50% at 40 Gy), bowel (maximal dose, <50 Gy; <35% of small bowel receiving ≥35 Gy), kidneys (maximal dose, 45 Gy; <35% at 16 Gy), rectum (maximal dose, <50 Gy; <40% of rectal volume receiving ≥40 Gy), and spinal cord (maximal dose, 40 Gy). Portelance et al. (57) used bladder (<50% at 40 Gy), colon and small intestine (<50% at 30 Gy), kidneys (<33% at 10 Gy), rectum (<50% at 30 Gy), and spinal cord (<5% at 45 Gy).

Toxicity and Outcomes

Salama et al. (61) reported their experience in treating 13 women with endometrial or cervical cancer with EF-IMRT. Grade ≥3 acute and late toxicity occurred in two patients. Gerszten et al. (62) did not observe any grade ≥3 acute GI or GU toxicity in 22 patients treated with EFRT, but outcomes and late toxicity data for these patients are not yet available. Beriwal et al. (63) treated 36 women with paraaortic nodal involvement or other high-risk features and found 65% overall survival at 2 years with low rates of acute grade ≥3 GI and GU toxicity. Grade ≥3 hematologic toxicity occurred in 28% of patients, which is an improvement from conventional treatment in some studies which reported grade ≥3 hematologic toxicity

of up 80%. Late toxicity in EF-IMRT studies ranges from 5 to 10%, compared with 10 to 40% with conventional treatment.

Du et al. (64) conducted a randomized trial of paraaortic IMRT compared with conventional paraaortic treatment in 60 patients with positive paraaortic nodes. All patients received conventional pelvic RT prior to paraaortic RT. They observed significantly higher 3-year survival (36.4 vs. 15.6%, $p = .016$) and lower toxicity in the EF-IMRT group.

An additional advantage of EF-IMRT is the potential to decrease kidney dose in cervical cancer patients, who are receiving cisplatin, a nephrotoxic drug. In a group of 23 patients receiving paraaortic IMRT, Varlotto et al. (65) observed decreased creatinine clearance, but did not find any clinical signs of nephrotoxicity.

Jensen et al. recently analyzed 21 patients treated at the University of Chicago and University of California San Diego (UCSD) with concurrent weekly cisplatin and EF-IMRT (66). Median follow-up was 18 months. The 18-month rates of locoregional and distant failure were 10.0% (95% CI, 1.6–28.4) and 46.1% (95% CI, 22.6–66.7), respectively. Acute grade ≥3 GI, GU and hematologic toxicity occurred in 4, 0, and 12 patients, respectively. The 2-year cumulative incidence of late grade ≥3 GU toxicity was 4.8% (95% CI, 0.2–20.3). No patients experienced late grade ≥3 GI toxicity.

■ PELVIC-INGUINAL RT

Dosimetric Studies, Treatment Planning, and Delivery

IMRT plans for vulvar cancer have been found to decrease the mean volume of bladder, bowel, and rectum receiving >30 Gy compared with 3DCRT plans (67,68). Beriwal et al. (69) have described their IMRT technique in detail. Patients undergo CT simulation in the supine position using custom immobilization, with bolus and radio-opaque wire placement as appropriate. The CTV includes the bilateral external iliac, internal iliac, and inguinofemoral nodes, with a margin of 1 to 2 cm around the named vessel, plus the entire vulvar region. A margin of 1 cm around the vulva and gross tumor is used. The CTV extends superiorly to 2 cm below L5-S1. The CTV is expanded 1 cm to generate the PTV. Critical structures are the small bowel, bladder, rectum, and femoral heads. Typical input parameters for dynamic multi-leaf collimator-based IMRT planning are small bowel—V_{35} < 35%/max < 50 Gy; bladder—V_{40} < 40%/max < 50 Gy; and rectum—V_{40} < 40%/max < 50 Gy. The prescription dose is normalized to the 95% isodose line. IMRT plans are considered acceptable if (1) the volume of PTV receiving < 95% of the prescribed dose ($V_{95\%}$) is <5%; (2) the PTV $V_{110\%}$ is <10%; and (3) the PTV $V_{120\%}$ is <1%. IMRT is delivered with concurrent 5-fluorouracil (5-FU) and cisplatin in a hybrid hyperfractionation regimen, with 1.6 Gy BID × 10 fractions, followed by 1.8 Gy QD × 7 to 8 fractions, followed by a 10- to 14-day break, followed by 1.6 Gy BID × 10, for a total dose of 44.6 to 46.4 Gy. Gross disease is resected 6 to 8 weeks following chemoradiotherapy.

Toxicity and Outcomes

Preoperative RT is often used in women with locally advanced cancer of the vulva to shrink tumor and decrease surgical morbidity. Beriwal et al. (69) treated 18 women with preoperative IMRT and observed no grade ≥3 acute or late toxicity, compared with 32% of patients experiencing grade 4 mucocutaneous toxicity reported in larger series using conventional RT techniques (70). Clinical and pathological complete response after RT was comparable with studies using conventional techniques.

■ WHOLE-ABDOMINAL RT

Dosimetric Studies

The use of whole-abdominal RT for ovarian and locally advanced endometrial cancer has declined due to toxicities associated with conventional techniques. IMRT offers an alternative treatment option for these patients, who are at high risk for abdominal recurrence of disease, despite combination chemotherapy. Dosimetric planning studies have shown that IMRT can improve PTV coverage relative to conventional plans, while maintaining kidney dose constraints and decreasing dose to pelvic bones (71). Duthoy et al. (72) studied five ovarian cancer patients undergoing treatment with whole-abdominal IMAT. The authors observed improved PTV dose homogeneity compared with four-field plans. Whole-abdominal arc plans can achieve similar target coverage to

IMRT, and can be delivered in a shorter timeframe (~5 min for arc therapy compared with ~18 min for IMRT) (73).

Treatment Planning and Delivery

Mahantshetty et al. (73) described both fixed-field and arc IMRT techniques for whole-abdominal RT. A bladder-filling protocol of voiding followed by 500 to 1000 mL is used 45 min prior to CT simulation. Patients undergo CT simulation in the supine position with arms overhead. The simulation scan extends from midthorax to midthigh using 5 mm slice thickness. The abdominal CTV (CTV_{WAR}) includes the entire peritoneal cavity, including bowel and mesentery, liver capsule with surface of liver parenchyma, abdominal surface of the diaphragm, and anterolateral surfaces of the kidneys. The pelvic CTV (CTV_{PELVIS}) includes the pelvic lymph nodes, pouch of Douglas, and vaginal vault, and extends from L5-S1. The PTV_{WAR} is defined by applying a 1.5-cm margin superiorly and a 0.5-cm margin in all other directions; the PTV_{PELVIS} is defined by applying a 1.0-cm margin inferiorly and a 0.5-cm margin in all other directions.

A simultaneous integrated boost (SIB) technique is used, with 1 Gy per day delivered to PTV_{WAR} and 1.8 Gy per day delivered to PTV_{PELVIS}. The plan is normalized to the mean dose to PTV_{PELVIS}. Beam energies are 6 and/or 15 MV photons. Arc plans use a maximum dose rate of 600 MU/min and fixed-field plans use a fixed dose rate of 600 MU/min. Two isocenters are used, separated by 15 cm along the cranio–caudal axis (z), with alignment in x and y coordinates. There is 5 cm overlap between the upper and lower fields or arc. Fixed-field IMRT use 14 equally spaced coplanar beams with 0° collimator angle. Arc plans are optimized with 3 arcs: 2 of 360° and 1 of 280° excluding the posterior sector.

Critical structures are the kidneys, liver, bone marrow, bladder, rectum, and heart, excluding portions extending into the PTV. Planning objectives are (1) PTV $V_{90\%}$ > 95%; (2) PTV_{PELVIS} maximum dose to 2% of the volume ($D_{2\%}$) < 105% of the prescription dose; and (3) PTV_{PELVIS} $V_{107\%}$ < 1%. Normal tissue input constraints were not specified in this protocol. However, IMRT and arc plans were able to achieve good normal tissue sparing, with mean bone marrow dose < 23 Gy, bladder V_{40} < 58% and $D_{1\%}$ < 47 Gy, heart mean dose < 8 Gy and $D_{1\%}$ < 25

Gy, kidney mean dose < 16 Gy and V_{20} < 42%, liver V_{20} < 80% and $D_{1\%}$ < 30 Gy, and rectum V_{45} < 15% and $D_{1\%}$ < 47 Gy.

Toxicity and Outcomes

Outcomes studies for patients treated with whole-abdominal IMRT for ovarian cancer are limited. In a phase I trial, IMRT for ovarian cancer was reported to be feasible and well-tolerated (74–76), with all patients completing therapy. Three, one, and one patients experienced acute grade 3 leukopenia, thrombocytopenia, and diarrhea, respectively. Three patients developed adhesions which required surgery. Two-year actuarial disease-free survival and overall survival were 63 and 68%, respectively. A phase II whole-abdominal IMRT trial of 37 women with optimally debulked ovarian cancer is currently underway (77), but outcome data are not yet available.

■ NOVEL IMRT APPLICATIONS

Bone-Marrow-Sparing IMRT

Hematologic toxicity is a common acute complication of pelvic RT, particularly when combined with chemotherapy. A large proportion of the active bone marrow in the adult is located in the pelvis and lumbosacral spine, making it challenging to avoid when treating gynecologic malignancies. Bone-marrow-sparing IMRT plans can decrease bone marrow dose compared with conventional techniques (78,79), which may lead to decreased hematologic toxicity. Brixey et al. (80) initially reported significantly lower levels of hematologic toxicity in gynecologic patients treated with IMRT (31%) than historic controls treated with conventional RT (60%). V_{10} and V_{20} for bone marrow have been found to correlate with acute hematologic toxicity (81,82). Specifically, limiting V_{10} to <95% and V_{20} to <75% may decrease the likelihood of grade ≥3 leukopenia (83). While bone marrow dose constraints for extended-field IMRT patients are not well-established, V_{10} and V_{20} of both pelvic and lumbosacral bone marrow have also been found to correlate with leukopenia in this setting (84).

Bone-marrow-sparing IMRT is constrained by the large volume of pelvic bones to avoid, and the need to spare other normal tissues. One strategy to optimize bone-marrow-sparing IMRT is to use functional imaging to identify hematopoietically active subregions that have to be avoided during treatment planning. It is known that bone marrow is comprised of both yellow, fat-rich regions with low hematopoietic activity and red, fat-poor regions with high activity. Single photon emission computed tomography (SPECT), quantitative MRI, and PET have been used to identify active subregions, which may allow for treatment plans that result in increased bone-marrow-sparing (85–87). Recently, hematologic toxicity was found to be associated with increased dose specifically to bone marrow subregions that are active on ^{18}F-FDG-PET (88), suggesting that techniques designed to avoid active subregions could reduce hematologic toxicity. UCSD recently completed a phase I trial of functional bone-marrow-sparing IMRT, using a combination of quantitative MRI and FDG-PET to define active bone marrow subregions (Figure 3) (86). Thirty-one women were enrolled on the study, and 10 were treated with functional bone-marrow-sparing IMRT. Preliminary results indicate this technique is feasible, with approximately 36% relative reduction in acute hematologic toxicity compared with contemporary controls (personal communication).

IMRT as an Alternative to Brachytherapy

Multiple planning studies have investigated the potential of IMRT to achieve a dose distribution similar to brachytherapy (89–92). Chan et al. (89) compared dosimetry of 3DCRT and four-field box RT with IMRT boost dosimetry in 12 gynecological cancer patients who could not receive brachytherapy. The authors found improved conformity with IMRT plans and a reduction of 22 and 19% for the volume of rectum and bladder receiving the highest doses, respectively. Malhotra et al. (90) found that similar target dose could be delivered with IMRT and brachytherapy in cervical cancer patients, but due to the steep dose fall-off of brachytherapy, integral OAR doses with brachytherapy were lower. Aydogan et al. (92) compared IMRT with high dose rate (HDR) brachytherapy in 10 patients with endometrial cancer. They found that IMRT provided better dose uniformity and improved bladder and rectal sparing compared with HDR.

Studies comparing IMRT and brachytherapy have been criticized for using brachytherapy techniques that were not fully optimized. A study

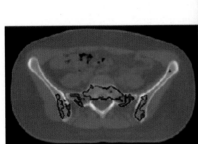
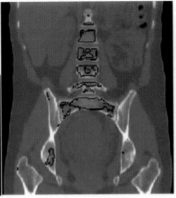
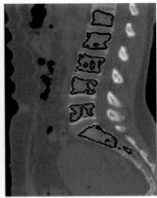

FIGURE 3 Overlay of segmented functional bone marrow on the simulation CT scan in the axial, coronal, and sagittal planes in a patient undergoing pelvic-paraaortic radiation therapy for cervical cancer. Functional bone marrow is defined by a combination of 18F-FDG-PET and quantitative MRI using iterative decomposition of water and fat with echo asymmetry and least-squares estimation (IDEAL-IQ). Thresholds are determined based on the mean standardized uptake value (18F-FDG-PET) and fat fraction (IDEAL-IQ) within the bone marrow.

comparing IMRT with high-tech brachytherapy found that for similar D_{2cc} and D_{1cc}, brachytherapy achieved higher D_{90} to the high- and intermediate-risk PTV compared with IMRT. Moreover, IMRT approximately doubled the total volume of tissue receiving >60 Gy (93).

IMRT as a concomitant boost to brachytherapy has also been evaluated. Assenholt et al. (94) evaluated applicator-guided IMRT boost combined with brachytherapy to improve coverage of large or topographically unfavorable tumors. IMRT was able to improve but did not replace the dose given by intracavitary brachytherapy in this study. Duan et al. (95) compared conventional brachytherapy versus optimized brachytherapy versus optimized brachytherapy with an IMRT boost. The authors found that optimized brachytherapy resulted in higher doses to OARs, and that HDR plus IMRT achieved better CTV coverage and adequate OAR sparing in cases where conventional brachytherapy dose was suboptimal.

Simultaneous Integrated Boost

IMRT can deliver different levels of dose to subregions of the CTV, allowing for macroscopic and microscopic disease areas to be treated to different doses within a single fraction (i.e., SIB). Several studies have evaluated SIB in cervical cancer patients. Kavanagh et al. (96) initially described their experience in seven patients in which tumor anatomy limited the deliverable brachytherapy dose. They delivered 1.8 Gy/fraction to the CTV and 2 to 2.2 Gy/fraction to the GTV and observed a complete response in all seven patients, with two patients experiencing acute grade 3 toxicity. Guerrero et al. (97) compared SIB with consecutive external beam and brachytherapy boost and found that SIB could provide better or equivalent tumor dose with improved normal tissue sparing. An advantage of SIB is that it decreases the overall treatment time for patients who would otherwise be treated with a sequential boost. However, inter-fraction tumor motion and regression need to be carefully taken into account when applying such techniques.

Stereotactic Body RT

Multiple case series have been published on SBRT for gynecologic cancers. For example, Choi et al. (98) used CyberKnife therapy of 33 to 45 Gy in three fractions to treat 30 patients with isolated paraaortic nodal recurrence. Overall survival and locoregional control at 4 years were 50 and 67%, respectively. Complications included grade ≥3 hematologic toxicity in five patients and a ureteral stricture in one patient at 20 months posttreatment. Mollà et al. (99) investigated SBRT in 16 women with gynecologic malignancies, as an alternative to brachytherapy. For postoperative patients, 14 Gy in two fractions was used, and 20 Gy in five fractions was used for patients treated definitively. There were no acute complications, but a grade 3 rectal complication occurred at 18 months. For further discussion on SBRT in the treatment of gynecologic cancers, including oligometastatic disease, the reader is referred to the review by Higginson et al. (100).

■ INTER- AND INTRAFRACTION MOTION

Concerns with IMRT for gynecologic malignancies are intra- and interfraction target motion and regression. Significant tumor regression occurs during treatment, and tumor volume may decrease to 50% of planning CT volume after a cumulative dose of 31 Gy has been delivered (101,102). In addition to decreasing in size over the course of treatment, tumors can also become more irregularly shaped.

A number of studies using interval imaging have shown significant interfraction motion during external beam RT (27–33,103), recommending planning margins from 10 to 40 mm to fully encompass the CTV for all fractions. Collen et al. (30) evaluated 10 patients with three times weekly megavoltage CT (MVCT) and found the largest motion to occur in the anterior/posterior and superior-inferior directions. They recommended anterior (A), posterior (P), right (R), left (L), superior (S), and inferior (I) margins around the uterus and cervix of 19, 19, 13, 13, 20, and 19 mm and 17, 12, 8, 9, 15, and 9 mm, respectively, to achieve 95% coverage. Van de bunt et al. (29) evaluated 20 patients with weekly MRI and recommended similar CTV margins of 24, 17, 12, 16, 11, and 8 in the A, P, R, L, S, and I directions. A larger analysis of 50 women undergoing daily kilovoltage (kV) cone-beam CT (CBCT) found that planning margins of approximately 5, 10, and 15 mm around the lymph nodes, cervix, and uterus, would ensure 95% probability of CTV coverage throughout the course of external beam RT, if daily image-guided RT (IGRT) for bone matching is used (33).

Identifying factors that predict variations in interfraction motion could help to determine who is most likely to benefit from IGRT, but these factors are not yet well-established. Huh et al. (103) found that greater change during treatment was associated with age <60 years and tumor size >4 cm. Several studies have assessed the relationship of bladder and rectal filling to CTV movement. Buchali et al. (104) found that the uterus and cervix were displaced

superiorly, but not in the anterior/posterior or LR direction with bladder and rectal filling. Tyagi et al. (31) also reported superior displacement of the CTV with bladder and rectal filling and posterior displacement with rectal filling.

Interfraction motion for postoperative patients has also been studied. Jhingran et al. (105) observed motion of seeds placed in the vaginal apex of 24 postoperative patients and found median maximal displacement of 0.59, 1.46, and 1.2 cm in the LR, anterior/posterior, and SI directions. They also evaluated consistency of bladder volumes in patients being treated on a full-bladder protocol and found that despite instructions, patients were unable to maintain consistent bladder filling, which is similar to reports from other studies using full-bladder protocol (106). A recent study of 11 postoperative cervical and endometrial cancer patients, using no bladder- or rectal-filling protocol, found average vaginal cuff movement of 1.6 cm, with a maximum movement of 3.4 cm on daily MVCT imaging (107). Based on these findings, uniform 1 cm margins would have resulted in 53% chance of vaginal cuff being outside the CTV on any given fraction. Another recent study of 22 postoperative cervical and endometrial cancer patients also imaged with daily MVCT observed maximum center of mass displacement of 2.6 cm. They concluded that uniform margins of 16 mm or directional margins of 3.1 mm along the right–left axis, 9.5 mm along the superoinferior axis, and of 12.1 mm along the anterior/posterior axis would account for 95% of observed motion (108).

Intrafraction motion has not been as widely studied, but considerable CTV motion can occur even during a 16-min simulated treatment, with one study reporting a maximal displacement of 9.9 mm in 90% of observed fractions (109). These authors found that intrafraction soft tissue registration could correct for this motion, but bone registration did not provide an advantage over no registration. Haripotepornkul et al. (32) also studied intrafraction motion and reported that while mean motion of the cervix (as measured by implanted seed motion) was only 2 to 4 mm, maximum motion was as high as 15 mm.

Studies calculating the actual dose delivered to CTV have generally shown adequate target coverage despite organ motion. Tyagi et al. (31) found that uniform 15-mm margins would not include portions of the CTV in 32% of daily images, but on average, the volume missed was small (<21 cc). A study of 10 patients immobilized with a small bowel displacement system found that CTV was adequately covered over the course of treatment with 15 mm uniform planning margins, based on CT repeated three times during treatment (110). Lim et al. (111) compared accumulated dose for 20 patients using four-field box, large-margin (10 mm) plans, and small-margin (5 mm) plans. Even with the small margin, they found that the GTV received >95% of the prescription dose in all patients, and in all but one patient, the CTV also received >95% of the prescription dose.

Several options exist to address the issue of interfraction motion. The simplest is to increase the CTV to PTV margins to ensure greater target coverage, but the addition of even a few millimeters to a uniform planning margin has been shown to significantly increase the dose to OARs (112). Another strategy would be to identify the factors that predict for a greater degree of motion (body mass index, tumor size, etc). Studies to date have not shown any such factors that could be reliably used in treatment planning, but pretreatment variable bladder-filling scans have been found to be potentially useful in predicting position change during treatment (113). ITV is another method to encompass potential organ motion during treatment planning. The ITV is generated by contouring the CTV on a full-bladder scan and an empty bladder scan, then fusing the two CTVs. A margin is then added to this ITV to create the PTV (114). Because the ITV takes into account the change in position of the CTV between full and empty bladder scans, the margin added may be smaller than if a single CT was used for treatment planning.

Adaptive RT is an alternative strategy to account for tumor motion and change. Replanning during treatment or selecting the best daily plan from a series of preplanned plans may allow for adequate or better coverage with smaller margins. Kerkhof et al. (115) compared preplanning with weekly replanning for 11 cervical cancer patients using a 10- to 15-mm CTV to PTV margin for the preplan and a 4-mm margin for the weekly replan. Using these margins, they found that organ volume overlapping with the PTV decreased from 53 to 11% for the bladder, 57 to 13% for the rectum, and 63 to 13% for the sigmoid colon. Stewart et al. (116) compared weekly replanning with no replanning using 3 mm margins and found that without replanning, only 73% of patients had acceptable CTV coverage based on weekly MRI. Van de Bunt et al. (102) also evaluated replanning

once during treatment and found that while dose to rectum decreased for all patients, dose to bladder and bowel only decreased in a subset of patients with significant tumor regression.

Challenges in adaptive RT using preplanning or replanning strategies include the significant amount of physician and dosimetrist time needed to generate an IMRT plan. Autocontouring programs, if developed, could assist in generating CTV on the daily or weekly image. Semiautomated contouring programs have been evaluated and found to have fair level of agreement with manual contours, but this technology is still investigational (117).

■ CONCLUSIONS AND FUTURE DIRECTIONS

One concern regarding IMRT in the treatment of gynecologic malignancies is the potential to increase second cancers due to increased integral tissue dose. A study of radiation-induced secondary malignancies found that the largest portion occurred in the marginal zone of the treated area and that 43% of second tumors occurred in areas receiving doses of <6 Gy (118). Studies have estimated IMRT could result in a 25% increase in the relative risk for second cancers (119). However, because the risk of secondary malignancy is relatively low after RT, this translates into only a small change in absolute risk. Long-term data evaluating the effect of IMRT on the risk of secondary cancers are needed.

Initial studies of IMRT for treatment of gynecologic cancer have shown favorable rates of toxicity and disease outcomes compared conventional techniques. Currently, however, there is limited prospective data and long-term follow-up. A randomized trial of IMRT for stage IIB cervical cancer is ongoing at Tata Memorial Hospital in Mumbai, India (120). The INTERTECC trial is an international multicenter phase II/III trial of IMRT in cervical cancer that will begin accrual in late 2011 or early 2012 (13). Finally, the RTOG is currently developing a randomized phase II trial in postoperative cervical and endometrial cancer with patient-reported outcomes as a primary endpoint. Hopefully, these studies will help establish the effects of IMRT on toxicity, disease control, and quality of life, relative to conventional techniques, and support its use in routine clinical practice.

■ REFERENCES

1. Green J, Kirwan J, Tierney J, et al. Concomitant chemo-therapy and radiation therapy for cancer of the uterine cervix. *Cochrane Database Syst Rev.* 2005;3:CD002225.

2. Baxter NN, Habermann EB, Tepper JE, et al. Risk of pelvic fractures in older women following pelvic irradiation. *JAMA.* 2005;294:2587–2593.

3. Greimel E, Thiel I, Peintinger F, Cegnar I, Pongratz E. Prospective assessment of quality of life of female cancer patients. *Gynecol Oncol.* 2002;85:140–147.

4. Mell LK, Mehrotra AK, Mundt AJ. Intensity-modulated radiation therapy use in the U.S., 2004. *Cancer.* 2005;104:1296–1303.

5. Roeske JC, Lujan A, Rotmensch J, et al. Intensity-modulated whole pelvic radiation therapy in patients with gynecologic malignancies. *Int J Radiat Oncol Biol Phys.* 2000;48:1613–1621.

6. Heron DE, Gerszten K, Selvaraj RN, et al. Conventional 3D conformal versus intensity-modulated radiotherapy for the adjuvant treatment of gynecologic malignancies: A comparative dosimetric study of dose-volume histograms. *Gynecol Oncol.* 2003;91:39–45.

7. Guo S, Ennis R, Bhatia S, et al. Assessment of nodal target definition and dosimetry using three different techniques: implications for re-defining the optimal pelvic field in endometrial cancer. *Radiat Oncol.* 2010;5:59.

8. Yang R, Xu S, Jiang W, et al. Dosimetric comparison of postoperative whole pelvic radiotherapy for endometrial cancer using three-dimensional conformal radiotherapy, intensity-modulated radiotherapy, and helical tomother-apy. *Acta Oncologica.* 2010;49:230–236.

9. Cozzi L, Dinshaw KA, Shrivastava SK, et al. A treatment planning study comparing volumetric arc modulation with RapidArc and fixed field IMRT for cervix uteri radiotherapy. *Radiother Oncol.* 2008;89:180–191.

10. Wong E, D'Souza DP, Chen JZ, et al. Intensity-modulated arc therapy for treatment of high-risk endometrial malignancies. *Int J Radiat Oncol Biol Phys.* 2005;61:830–841.

11. Macdonald DM, Lin LL, Biehl K, et al. Combined intensity-modulated radiation therapy and brachytherapy in the treatment of cervical cancer. *Int J Radiat Oncol Biol Phys.* 2008;71:618–624.

12. Cilla S, Macchia G, Digesù C, et al. 3D-Conformal versus intensity-modulated postoperative radiotherapy of vaginal vault: a dosimetric comparison. *Med Dosim.* 2010;35:135–142.

13. Jensen L, Mahantshetty U, Shi M, et al. Survey of IMRT practices in centers participating in the international evaluation of radiotherapy technology effectiveness in cervical cancer (INTERTECC) trial (abstr.) *Int J Radiat Oncol Biol Phys.* 2011;81:S457–S458.

14. Adli M, Mayr NA, Kaiser HS, et al. Does prone positioning reduce small bowel dose in pelvic radiation with intensity-modulated radiotherapy for gynecologic cancer? *Int J Radiat Oncol Biol Phys.* 2003;57:230–238.

15. Stromberger C, Kom Y, Kawgan-Kagan M, et al. Intensity-modulated radiotherapy in patients with cervical cancer. An intra-individual comparison of prone and supine positioning. *Radiat Oncol.* 2010;5:63.

16. Huh SJ, Kang MK, Han Y. Small bowel displacement system-assisted intensity-modulated radiotherapy for cervical cancer. *Gynecol Oncol.* 2004;93:400–406.

17. Beriwal S, Jain SK, Heron DE, et al. Dosimetric and toxicity comparison between prone and supine position IMRT for endometrial cancer. *Int J Radiat Oncol Biol Phys.* 2007;67:485–489.

18. Haslam JJ, Lujan AE, Mundt AJ, et al. Setup errors in patients treated with intensity-modulated whole pelvic radiation therapy for gynecological malignancies. *Med Dosim.* 2005;30:36–42.

19. Gaffney DK, Du Bois A, Narayan K, et al. Practice patterns of radiotherapy in cervical cancer among member groups of the Gynecologic Cancer Intergroup (GCIG). *Int J Radiat Oncol Biol Phys.* 2007;68:485–490.

20. Mitchell DG, Snyder B, Coakley F, et al. Early invasive cervical cancer: tumor delineation by magnetic resonance imaging, computed tomography, and clinical examination, verified by pathologic results, in the ACRIN 6651/GOG 183 Intergroup study. *J Clin Oncol.* 2006;24:5687–5694.

21. Haie-Meder C, Mazeron R, Magné N. Clinical evidence on PET-CT for radiation therapy planning in cervix and endometrial cancers. *Radiother Oncol.* 2010;96:351–355.

22. Dehdashti F, Grigsby PW, Lewis JS, et al. Assessing tumor hypoxia in cervical cancer by PET with 60Cu-labeled diacetyl-bis(N4-methylthiosemicarbazone). *J Nucl Med.* 2008;49:201–205.

23. Small W, Jr., Mell LK, Anderson P, et al. Consensus guidelines for delineation of clinical target volume for intensity-modulated pelvic radiotherapy in postoperative treatment of endometrial and cervical cancer. *Int J Radiat Oncol Biol Phys.* 2008;71:428–434.

24. Lim K, Small W, Jr., Portelance L, et al. Consensus guidelines for delineation of clinical target volume for intensity-modulated pelvic radiotherapy for the definitive treatment of cervix cancer. *Int J Radiat Oncol Biol Phys.* 2011;79:348–355.

25. Guidelines for the delineation of the CTV in postoperative pelvic RT. Available at: http://www.rtog.org/CoreLab/ContouringAtlases/GYN.aspx. Accessed July 31, 2011.

26. *Contouring guidelines for INTERTECC trial.* Available at: http://radonc.ucsd.edu/RESEARCH/IRTOC/Pages/videos.aspx. Accessed July 31, 2011.

27. Chan P, Dinniwell R, Haider MA, et al. Inter- and intra-fractional tumor and organ movement in patients with cervical cancer undergoing radiotherapy: A cinematic-MRI point-of-interest study. *Int J Radiat Oncol Biol Phys.* 2008;70:1507–1515.

28. Kaatee RSJP, Olofsen MJJ, Verstraate MBJ, et al. Detection of organ movement in cervix cancer patients using a fluoroscopic electronic portal imaging device and radiopaque markers. *Int J Radiat Oncol Biol Phys.* 2002;54:576–583.

29. van de Bunt L, Jürgenliemk-Schulz IM, de Kort GAP, et al. Motion and deformation of the target volumes during IMRT for cervical cancer: what margins do we need? *Radiother Oncol.* 2008;88:233–240.

30. Collen C, Engels B, Duchateau M, et al. Volumetric imaging by megavoltage computed tomography for assessment of internal organ motion during radiotherapy for cervical cancer. *Int J Radiat Oncol Biol Phys.* 2010;77:1590–1595.

31. Tyagi N, Lewis JH, Yashar CM, et al. Daily online cone beam computed tomography to assess interfractional motion in patients with intact cervical cancer. *Int J Radiat Oncol Biol Phys.* 2011;80:273–280.

32. Haripotepornkul N, Nath S, Scanderbeg D, et al. Evaluation of intra- and inter-fraction movement of the cervix during intensity modulated radiation therapy. *Radiother Oncol.* 2011;98:5.

33. Khan A, Jensen LG, Sun S, et al. Optimized planning target volume for intact cervical cancer. *Int J Radiat Oncol Biol Phys.* 2011; in press.

34. Roeske JC, Bonta D, Mell LK, et al. A dosimetric analysis of acute gastrointestinal toxicity in women receiving intensity-modulated whole-pelvic radiation therapy. *Radiother Oncol.* 2003;69:201–207.

35. Simpson DS, Song WY, Rose BS, et al. Normal tissue complication probability analysis of acute gastrointestinal toxicity in cervical cancer patients undergoing intensity modulated radiation therapy and concurrent cisplatin (abstr.). *Int J Radiat Oncol Biol Phys.* 2010; 78:S141–S142.

36. Kavanagh BD, Pan CC, Dawson LA, et al. Radiation dose-volume effects in the stomach and small bowel. *Int J Radiat Oncol Biol Phys.* 2010;76:S101–S107.

37. Mundt AJ, Roeske JC, Lujan AE, et al. Initial clinical experience with intensity-modulated whole-pelvis radiation therapy in women with gynecologic malignancies. *Gynecol Oncol.* 2001;82:456–463.

38. Mundt AJ, Lujan AE, Rotmensch J, et al. Intensity-modulated whole pelvic radiotherapy in women with gynecologic malignancies. *Int J Radiat Oncol Biol Phys.* 2002;52:1330–1337.

39. Mundt AJ, Mell LK, Roeske JC. Preliminary analysis of chronic gastrointestinal toxicity in gynecology patients treated with intensity-modulated whole pelvic radiation therapy. *Int J Radiat Oncol Biol Phys.* 2003;56:1354–1360.

40. Knab BR, Roeske JC, Mehta N, Sutton H, Mundt AJ. Outcome of endometrial cancer patients treated with adjuvant intensity modulated pelvic radiation therapy (abstr.). *Int J Radiat Oncol Biol Phys.* 2004;60:S303–S304.

41. Beriwal S, Jain SK, Heron DE, et al. Clinical outcome with adjuvant treatment of endometrial carcinoma using intensity-modulated radiation therapy. *Gynecol Oncol.* 2006;102:195–199.

42. Tierney RM, Powell MA, Mutch DG, et al. Acute toxicity of postoperative IMRT and chemotherapy for endometrial cancer. *Radiat Med.* 2007;25:439–445.

43. Bouchard M, Nadeau S, Gingras L, et al. Clinical outcome of adjuvant treatment of endometrial cancer using aperture-based intensity-modulated radiotherapy. *Int J Radiat Oncol Biol Phys.* 2008;71:1343–1350.

44. Chen M-F, Tseng C-J, Tseng C-C, et al. Clinical outcome in posthysterectomy cervical cancer patients treated with concurrent cisplatin and intensity-modulated pelvic radiotherapy: comparison with conventional radiotherapy. *Int J Radiat Oncol Biol Phys.* 2007;67:1438–1444.

45. Hasselle MD, Rose BS, Kochanski JD, et al. Clinical outcomes of intensity-modulated pelvic radiation therapy for carcinoma of the cervix. *Int J Radiat Oncol Biol Phys.* 2010;80:1436–1445.

46. Jhingran A, Winter K, Portelance L, et al. A phase ii study of intensity modulated radiation therapy (IMRT) to the pelvic for post-operative patients with endometrial carcinoma (RTOG 0418) (abstr.). *Int J Radiat Oncol Biol Phys.* 2008;72:S16–S17.

47. Portelance L, Winter K, Jhingran A, et al. Post-operative pelvic intensity modulated radiation therapy (IMRT) with chemotherapy for patients with cervical carcinoma/ RTOG 0418 phase II study (abstr.). *Int J Radiat Oncol Biol Phys.* 2009;75:S640–S641.

48. Schwarz JK, Wahab S, Grigsby PW, et al. prospective phase I-II trial of helical tomotherapy with or without chemotherapy for postoperative cervical cancer patients. *Int J Radiat Oncol Biol Phys.* 2010;PMID:20932657.

49. Kidd EA, Siegel BA, Dehdashti F, et al. Clinical outcomes of definitive intensity-modulated radiation therapy with fluorodeoxyglucose-positron emission tomography simulation in patients with locally advanced cervical cancer. *Int J Radiat Oncol Biol Phys.* 2010;77:1085–1091.

50. Chen CC, Lin JC, Jan JS, Ho SC, Wang L. Definitive intensity-modulated radiation therapy with concurrent chemotherapy for patients with locally advanced cervical cancer. *Gynecol Oncol.* 2011;122:9–13.

51. Peters WA III, Liu PY, Barrett RJ II, et al. Concurrent chemo-therapy and pelvic radiation therapy compared with pelvic radiation therapy alone as adjuvant therapy after radical surgery in high-risk early-stage cancer of the cervix. *J Clin Oncol.* 2000;18:1606–1613.

52. Nugent EK, Case AS, Hoff JT, et al. Chemoradiation in locally advanced cervical carcinoma: An analysis of cisplatin dosing and other clinical prognostic factors. *Gynecol Oncol.* 2010;116:438–441.

53. Hsieh C, Wei M, Lee H, et al. Whole pelvic helical tomotherapy for locally advanced cervical cancer: technical

implementation of IMRT with helical tomotherapy. *Radiat Oncol.* 2009;4:62.

54. Vera R, Eifel PJ, Jhingran A, Salepour M. intensity-modulated radiation therapy (IMRT) in the treatment of carcinoma of the vagina (abstr.). *Int J Radiat Oncol Biol Phys.* 2007;69:S396.

55. Ahmed RS, Kim RY, Duan J, et al. IMRT dose escalation for positive para-aortic lymph nodes in patients with locally advanced cervical cancer while reducing dose to bone marrow and other organs at risk. *Int J Radiat Oncol Biol Phys.* 2004;60:505–512.

56. Hermesse J, Devillers M, Deneufbourg J-M, et al. Can intensity-modulated radiation therapy of the paraaortic region overcome the problems of critical organ tolerance? *Strahlenther Onkol.* 2005;181:185–190.

57. Portelance L, Chao KSC, Grigsby PW, et al. Intensity-modulated radiation therapy (IMRT) reduces small bowel, rectum, and bladder doses in patients with cervical cancer receiving pelvic and para-aortic irradiation. *Int J Radiat Oncol Biol Phys.* 2001;51:261–266.

58. Lian J, Mackenzie M, Joseph K, et al. Assessment of extended-field radiotherapy for stage iiic endometrial cancer using three-dimensional conformal radiotherapy, intensity-modulated radiotherapy, and helical tomotherapy. *Int J Radiat Oncol Biol Phys.* 2008;70:935–943.

59. Mutic S, Malyapa RS, Grigsby PW, et al. PET-guided IMRT for cervical carcinoma with positive para-aortic lymph nodes—a dose-escalation treatment planning study. *Int J Radiat Oncol Biol Phys.* 2003;55:28–35.

60. Esthappan J, Chaudhari S, Santanam L, et al. Prospective clinical trial of positron emission tomography/computed tomography image-guided intensity-modulated radiation therapy for cervical carcinoma with positive para-aortic lymph nodes. *Int J Radiat Oncol Biol Phys.* 2008;72:1134–1139.

61. Salama JK, Mundt AJ, Roeske J, et al. Preliminary outcome and toxicity report of extended-field, intensity-modulated radiation therapy for gynecologic malignancies. *Int J Radiat Oncol Biol Phys.* 2006;65:1170–1176.

62. Gerszten K, Colonello K, Heron DE, et al. Feasibility of concurrent cisplatin and extended field radiation therapy (EFRT) using intensity-modulated radiotherapy (IMRT) for carcinoma of the cervix. *Gynecol Oncol.* 2006;102:182–188.

63. Beriwal S, Gan GN, Heron DE, et al. Early clinical outcome with concurrent chemotherapy and extended-field, intensity-modulated radiotherapy for cervical cancer. *Int J Radiat Oncol Biol Phys.* 2007;68:166–171.

64. Du X, Sheng X, Jiang T, et al. Intensity-modulated radiation therapy versus para-aortic field radiotherapy to treat para-aortic lymph node metastasis in cervical cancer: Prospective study. *Croat Med J.* 2010;51:8.

65. Varlotto J, Gerszten K, Heron D, et al. The potential nephrotoxic effects of intensity modulated radiotherapy

delivered to the para-aortic area of women with gynecologic malignancies: preliminary results. *Am J Clin Oncol.* 2006;29:8.

66. Jensen LG, Hasselle MD, Rose BS, et al. Outcomes for cervical cancer patients treated with extended field intensity-modulated radiation therapy and concurrent cisplatin (abstr.) *Int J Radiat Oncol Biol Phys.* 2011;81:S452–S453.

67. Beriwal S, Heron DE, Kim H, et al. Intensity-modulated radiotherapy for the treatment of vulvar carcinoma: A comparative dosimetric study with early clinical outcome. *Int J Radiat Oncol Biol Phys.* 2006;64:1395–1400.

68. Moran MS, Castrucci WA, Ahmad M, et al. Clinical utility of the modified segmental boost technique for treatment of the pelvis and inguinal nodes. *Int J Radiat Oncol Biol Phys.* 2010;76:1026–1036.

69. Beriwal S, Coon D, Heron DE, et al. Preoperative intensity-modulated radiotherapy and chemotherapy for locally advanced vulvar carcinoma. *Gynecol Oncol.* 2008;109:291–295.

70. Montana GS, Thomas GM, Moore DH, et al. Preoperative chemo-radiation for carcinoma of the vulva with N2/N3 nodes: A gynecologic oncology group study. *Int J Radiat Oncol Biol Phys.* 2000;48:1007–1013.

71. Hong L, Alektiar K, Chui C, et al. IMRT of large fields: Whole-abdomen irradiation. *Int J Radiat Oncol Biol Phys.* 2002;54:278–289.

72. Duthoy W, De Gersem W, Vergote K, et al. Whole abdominopelvic radiotherapy (WAPRT) using intensity-modulated arc therapy (IMAT): First clinical experience. *Int J Radiat Oncol Biol Phys.* 2003;57:1019–1032.

73. Mahantshetty U, Jamema S, Engineer R, et al. Whole abdomen radiation therapy in ovarian cancers: A comparison between fixed beam and volumetric arc based intensity modulation. *Radiat Oncol.* 2010;5:106.

74. Jensen AD, Nill S, Rochet N, et al. Whole-abdominal IMRT for advanced ovarian carcinoma: Planning issues and feasibility. *Physica Medica.* 2011;27:194–202.

75. Rochet N, Jensen A, Sterzing F, et al. Adjuvant whole abdominal intensity modulated radiotherapy (IMRT) for high risk stage FIGO III patients with ovarian cancer (OVAR-IMRT-01)—Pilot trial of a phase I/II study: Study protocol. *BMC Cancer.* 2007;7:227.

76. Rochet N, Sterzing F, Jensen AD, et al. Intensity-modulated whole abdominal radiotherapy after surgery and carboplatin/taxane chemotherapy for advanced ovarian cancer: Phase I study. *Int J Radiat Oncol Biol Phys.* 2010;76:1382–1389.

77. Rochet N, Kieser M, Sterzing F, et al. Phase II study evaluating consolidation whole abdominal intensity-modulated radiotherapy (IMRT) in patients with advanced ovarian cancer stage FIGO III—The OVAR-IMRT-02 Study. *BMC Cancer.* 2011;11.

78. Mell LK, Tiryaki H, Ahn K-H, et al. Dosimetric comparison of bone marrow-sparing intensity-modulated radiotherapy

versus conventional techniques for treatment of cervical cancer. *Int J Radiat Oncol Biol Phys.* 2008;71:1504–1510.

79. Lujan AE, Mundt AJ, Yamada SD, et al. Intensity-modulated radiotherapy as a means of reducing dose to bone marrow in gynecologic patients receiving whole pelvic radiotherapy. *Int J Radiat Oncol Biol Phys.* 2003;57:516–521.

80. Brixey CJ, Roeske JC, Lujan AE, et al. Impact of intensity-modulated radiotherapy on acute hematologic toxicity in women with gynecologic malignancies. *Int J Radiat Oncol Biol Phys.* 2002;54:1388–1396.

81. Mell LK, Kochanski JD, Roeske JC, et al. Dosimetric predictors of acute hematologic toxicity in cervical cancer patients treated with concurrent cisplatin and intensity-modulated pelvic radiotherapy. *Int J Radiat Oncol Biol Phys.* 2006;66:1356–1365.

82. Albuquerque K, Giangreco D, Morrison C, et al. Radiation-related predictors of hematologic toxicity after concurrent chemoradiation for cervical cancer and implications for bone marrow-sparing pelvic IMRT. *Int J Radiat Oncol Biol Phys.* 2011;79:1043–1047.

83. Rose BS, Aydogan B, Liang Y, et al. Normal tissue complication probability modeling of acute hematologic toxicity in cervical cancer patients treated with chemoradiotherapy. *Int J Radiat Oncol Biol Phys.* 2011;79:800–807.

84. Rose BS, Nath SK, Manoj S, et al. Correlation between bone marrow dose and acute hematologic toxicity in cervical cancer patients treated with chemoradiotherapy: implications for extended-field intensity modulated radiation therapy (abstr.). *Int J Radiat Oncol Biol Phys.* 2010;78:S400.

85. Roeske JC, Lujan A, Reba RC, et al. Incorporation of SPECT bone marrow imaging into intensity modulated whole-pelvic radiation therapy treatment planning for gynecologic malignancies. *Radiother Oncol.* 2005;77:11–17.

86. Mell LK, Liang Y, Bydder M, et al. Functional MRI-guided bone marrow-sparing intensity modulated radiotherapy for pelvic malignancies. *Int J Radiat Oncol Biol Phys.* 2009;75:S121.

87. McGuire SM, Menda Y, Ponto LL, Gross B, Juweid M, Bayouth JE. A methodology for incorporating functional bone marrow sparing in IMRT planning for pelvic radiation therapy. *Radiother Oncol.* 2011;99:49–54.

88. Rose BS, Liang Y, Lau SK, et al. Correlation between radiation dose to 18F-FDG-PET defined active bone marrow sub-regions and acute hematologic toxicity in cervical cancer patients treated with chemoradiotherapy. *Int J Radiat Oncol Biol Phys.* 2011; in press.

89. Chan P, Yeo I, Perkins G, et al. Dosimetric comparison of intensity-modulated, conformal, and four-field pelvic radiotherapy boost plans for gynecologic cancer: A retrospective planning study. *Radiat Oncol.* 2006;1:10.

90. Malhotra H, Avadhani S, DeBoer S, et al. Duplicating a tandem and ovoids distribution with intensity-modulated radiotherapy: a feasibility study. *J Appl Clin Med Phys.* 2007;8:8.

91. Low DA, Grigsby PW, Dempsey JF, et al. Applicator-guided intensity-modulated radiation therapy. *Int J Radiat Oncol Biol Phys.* 2002;52:1400–1406.

92. Aydogan B, Mundt AJ, Smith BD, et al. A dosimetric analysis of intensity-modulated radiation therapy (IMRT) as an alternative to adjuvant high-dose-rate (HDR) brachytherapy in early endometrial cancer patients. *Int J Radiat Oncol Biol Phys.* 2006;65:266–273.

93. Georg D, Kirisits C, Hillbrand M, et al. Image-guided radiotherapy for cervix cancer: High-tech external beam therapy versus high-tech brachytherapy. *Int J Radiat Oncol Biol Phys.* 2008;71:1272–1278.

94. Assenholt MS, Petersen B, Jr., Nielsen SrK, et al. A dose planning study on applicator guided stereotactic IMRT boost in combination with 3D MRI based brachytherapy in locally advanced cervical cancer. *Acta Oncologica.* 2008;47:1337–1343.

95. Duan J, Kim RY, Elassal S, et al. Conventional high-dose-rate brachytherapy with concomitant complementary IMRT boost: A novel approach for improving cervical tumor dose coverage. *Int J Radiat Oncol Biol Phys.* 2008;71:765–771.

96. Kavanagh BD, Schefter TE, Wu Q, et al. Clinical application of intensity-modulated radiotherapy for locally advanced cervical cancer. *Semin Radiat Oncol.* 2002;12:260–271.

97. Guerrero M, Li XA, Ma L, et al. Simultaneous integrated intensity-modulated radiotherapy boost for locally advanced gynecological cancer: radiobiological and dosimetric considerations. *Int J Radiat Oncol Biol Phys.* 2005;62:933–939.

98. Choi CW, Cho ÇK, Yoo SY, et al. Image-guided stereotactic body radiation therapy in patients with isolated para-aortic lymph node metastases from uterine cervical and corpus cancer. *Int J Radiat Oncol Biol Phys.* 2009;74:147–153.

99. Mollà M, Escude L, Nouet P, et al. Fractionated stereotactic radiotherapy boost for gynecologic tumors: an alternative to brachytherapy? *Int J Radiat Oncol Biol Phys.* 2005;62:118–124.

100. Higginson DS, Morris DE, Jones EL, Clarke-Pearson D, Varia MA. Stereotactic body radiotherapy (SBRT): Technological innovation and application in gynecologic oncology. *Gynecol Oncol.* 2011;120:404–412.

101. Lee CM, Shrieve DC, Gaffney DK. Rapid involution and mobility of carcinoma of the cervix. *Int J Radiat Oncol Biol Phys.* 2004;58:625–630.

102. van de Bunt L, van der Heide UA, Ketelaars M, et al. Conventional, conformal, and intensity-modulated radiation therapy treatment planning of external beam radiotherapy for cervical cancer: The impact of tumor regression. *Int J Radiat Oncol Biol Phys.* 2006;64:189–196.

103. Huh SJ, Park W, Han Y. Interfractional variation in position of the uterus during radical radiotherapy for cervical cancer. *Radiother Oncol.* 2004;71:73–79.

104. Buchali A, Koswig S, Dinges S, et al. Impact of the filling status of the bladder and rectum on their integral dose distribution and the movement of the uterus in the treatment planning of gynaecological cancer. *Radiother Oncol.* 1999;52:29–34.

105. Jhingran A, Salehpour M, Sam M, Levy L, Eifel PJ. Vaginal motion and bladder and rectal volumes during pelvic intensity-modulated radiation therapy after hysterectomy. *Int J Radiat Oncol Biol Phys.* 2011; PMID: 21093170.

106. Ahmad R, Hoogeman MS, Quint S, et al. Inter-fraction bladder filling variations and time trends for cervical cancer patients assessed with a portable 3-dimensional ultrasound bladder scanner. *Radiother Oncol.* 2008;89:172–179.

107. Ma DJ, Michaletz-Lorenz M, Goddu SM, et al. Magnitude of interfractional vaginal cuff movement: implications for external irradiation. *Int J Radiat Oncol Biol Phys.* 2011; PMID: 21703780.

108. Harris EE, Latifi K, Rusthoven C, et al. Assessment of organ motion in postoperative endometrial and cervical cancer patients treated with intensity-modulated radiation therapy. *Int J Radiat Oncol Biol Phys.* 2011; PMID: 21640508.

109. Kerkhof EM, van der Put RW, Raaymakers BW, et al. Intrafraction motion in patients with cervical cancer: the benefit of soft tissue registration using MRI. *Radiother Oncol.* 2009;93:115–121.

110. Han Y, Shin EH, Huh SJ, et al. Interfractional dose variation during intensity-modulated radiation therapy for cervical cancer assessed by weekly CT evaluation. *Int J Radiat Oncol Biol Phys.* 2006;65:617–623.

111. Lim K, Kelly V, Stewart J, et al. Pelvic radiotherapy for cancer of the cervix: is what you plan actually what you deliver? *Int J Radiat Oncol Biol Phys.* 2009;74:304–312.

112. Ahamad A, D'Souza W, Salehpour M, et al. Intensity-modulated radiation therapy after hysterectomy: comparison with conventional treatment and sensitivity of the normal-tissue-sparing effect to margin size. *Int J Radiat Oncol Biol Phys.* 2005;62:1117–1124.

113. Ahmad R, Hoogeman MS, Bondar M, et al. Increasing treatment accuracy for cervical cancer patients using correlations between bladder-filling change and cervix-uterus displacements: Proof of principle. *Radiother Oncol.* 2011;98:340–346.

114. *RTOG 0418 Protocol.* Available at: http://www.rtog.org/ClinicalTrials/ProtocolTable/StudyDetails.aspx?study=0418. Accessed July 31, 2011.

115. Kerkhof EM, Raaymakers BW, van der Heide UA, et al. Online MRI guidance for healthy tissue sparing in patients with cervical cancer: An IMRT planning study. *Radiother Oncol.* 2008;88:241–249.

116. Stewart J, Lim K, Kelly V, et al. Automated weekly replanning for intensity-modulated radiotherapy of cervix cancer. *Int J Radiat Oncol Biol Phys.* 2010;78:350–358.

117. Wu DH, Shaffer AD, Thompson DM, et al. Iterative active deformational methodology for tumor delineation: Evaluation across radiation treatment stage and volume. *J Mag Res Imag.* 2008;28:1188–1194.

118. Dorr W, Hermann T. Second primary tumors after radiotherapy for malignancies. Treatment-related parameters. *Strahlenther Onkol.* 2002;178:6.

119. Zwahlen DR, Ruben JD, Jones P, et al. Effect of intensity-modulated pelvic radiotherapy on second cancer risk in the postoperative treatment of endometrial and cervical cancer. *Int J Radiat Oncol Biol Phys.* 2009;74:539–545.

120. *A trial comparing intensity modulated radiation therapy (IMRT) with conventional radiation therapy in stage IIB carcinoma cervix.* Available at: http://clinicaltrials.gov/ct2/show/NCT00193804. Accessed July 31, 2011.

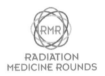

In-Room Image-Guided Radiation Therapy for Cervical Cancers

Mitch Kamrava[2], Loren K. Mell[1], and Catheryn M. Yashar[*1]
[1]*Department of Radiation Oncology, University of California, La Jolla, CA*
[2]*Department of Radiation Oncology, University of California, Los Angeles, CA*

■ ABSTRACT

The treatment of gynecologic malignancies is currently undergoing shift in management. Historically, treatment has been given with two to four fields with boundaries based on a bony anatomy. Technological advances have allowed for a more precise definition of targets and organs at risk. Intensity-modulated radiation therapy has allowed more conformal treatment of the target, with increased sparing of the normal tissues. With these advances, tumor identification and shrinkage and intra- and interfractional motion have been recognized as important factors and will affect both target and normal tissue doses. Image-guidance techniques for tumor detection, target definition, and in-room guidance are discussed with an emphasis on how these techniques improve the delivery of modern radiotherapy.

Keywords: IGRT, gynecologic, brachytherapy

■ INTRODUCTION

There has been a significant increase in the use of intensity-modulated radiation therapy (IMRT) for gynecologic malignancies over the past 10 years (1). Relative to conventional techniques, IMRT allows significantly lower doses to be delivered to the bowel, the rectum, the bladder, and the bone marrow. These reductions in turn are associated with decreased rates of acute and late gastrointestinal (GI), genitourinary (GU), and hematologic toxicities (2–7). Despite these improvements, widespread adoption of IMRT for gynecologic malignancies has been slow due to the increased complexities relative to three-dimensional (3D) planning in target delineation (8–10), patient setup (8,11), inter- and intrafraction motion, tumor regression during the course of treatment, and issues related to bladder and rectal filling (12–16).

Image-guided radiation therapy (IGRT) technologies are increasingly providing opportunities for improved target definition and daily localization, enabling greater sophistication in radiation delivery for gynecologic cancers. The combination of IGRT and more conformal radiation techniques promises to improve the therapeutic ratio of radiation by improving treatment accuracy while limiting toxicity to normal tissues. This chapter discusses

*Corresponding author, Rebecca and John Moores Cancer Center, Department of Radiation Oncology, 3855 Health Sciences Drive, San Diego, CA 92103
  E-mail address: cyashar@ucsd.edu

Radiation Medicine Rounds 2:3 (2011) 357–370.
DOI: 10.5003/2151–4208.2.3.357

image-guided target delineation of the clinical target volume (CTV), the planning target volume (PTV), issues related to daily treatment verification with IGRT, incorporation of positron emission tomography (PET), and magnetic resonance imaging (MRI) in radiation treatment planning, as well as future IGRT directions in gynecologic malignancies.

■ IMAGE-GUIDED CTV TARGET DELINEATION FOR EXTERNAL BEAM RADIATION THERAPY

Traditional "four-field box" pelvic radiation field borders are based on bony landmarks. The bony pelvis defines the lateral field edge on the anterior/posterior fields. The anterior border on the lateral fields is defined by the pubic symphysis and the posterior border is defined by the presacral space. Treatment based on these landmarks has resulted in excellent tumor control and acceptable toxicity. However, these landmarks are only a surrogate for the CTV and do not allow customization based on an individual's specific anatomy. With CT and MRI information we can now specifically define targets to help optimize target coverage and minimize normal tissue toxicity. To accomplish this, however, there needs to be agreement on what the specific targets are and how they should be contoured. The section below is a discussion of the consensus guidelines on CTV targets and delineation in patients with cervical cancer treated definitively and postoperatively.

Postoperative Cervix

Radiation Therapy Oncology Group (RTOG) 0418 is a prospective multi-institutional protocol investigating the use of IMRT in the postoperative setting for either cervical or endometrial cancer. In preparation for this study the RTOG established consensus guidelines for defining the CTV (9) (Figure 1). In the postoperative setting, the CTV targets should include: common iliac lymph nodes, external iliac lymph nodes, internal iliac lymph nodes, upper vagina, parametrial/paravaginal tissue, and presacral lymph nodes. Superiorly, the contours for the vessels should start 7 mm below the L4-L5 interspace. The inferior extent of the external iliac

lymph nodes should be at the femoral heads and the internal iliac lymph nodes should terminate in the paravaginal tissues at the level of the vaginal cuff. If presacral lymph nodes are included, the lymph node region anterior to the S1 and S2 regions should be contoured.

After the vessels have been contoured, a 7-mm expansion is suggested to ensure adequate coverage of the lymph nodes. The rationale for this expansion is based on the work by Taylor et al. who evaluated the location of pelvic lymph nodes in 20 women with gynecologic malignancies (12 cervical and 8 endometrial) by injecting intravenous iron oxide particles in conjunction with MRI (17). These investigators found that a modified 7-mm margin around the vessels served as a good surrogate to adequately encompass pelvic lymph nodes. This margin expansion was validated on a group of 10 women with gynecologic cancers who underwent MRI with and without intravenous iron oxide particles. By applying their suggested expansion the pelvic lymph nodes were fully covered in 99.5% of cases. There were only 4/741 (0.8%) identified lymph nodes that were not completely covered (two anterior external iliac nodes and two lateral external iliac nodes) (18).

Final clinical results from RTOG 0418 are pending; however, an abstract was presented in 2010, which included interim results on 106 postoperative patients (58 endometrial and 48 cervical cancers) treated to 50.4 Gy with or without cisplatin (19). Eighty-three patients had data available for

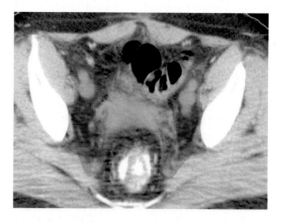

FIGURE 1 Consensus contours of the CTV on a CT scan for the postoperative treatment of cervical and endometrial carcinoma with IMRT.

analysis. Overall, 25% developed grade 2 or higher short-term bowel toxicity and no patients developed grade 4 bowel adverse events. In the patients treated with chemotherapy, there was minimal bone marrow toxicity with 80% of patients able to complete chemotherapy as planned (19). Long-term clinical and toxicity data utilizing the RTOG contouring guidelines are awaited, but early results are encouraging.

Intact Cervix

IMRT for the definitive treatment of intact cervical cancer has been reported by multiple groups; however, these studies used a wide range of CTV definitions (15,20–22). In an effort to standardize target definitions, the RTOG recently published IMRT consensus guidelines for intact cervix (Figure 2) (10). The nodal CTV should include the common iliac, internal iliac, external iliac, obturator, and presacral lymph nodes. The primary CTV should include the gross tumor volume (GTV), cervix (if not already included in the GTV), the entire uterus, parametria, ovaries, and vaginal tissues. The guidelines also provide specific details about the borders of the parametria. Superiorly, it should be bounded by the top of the fallopian tube/broad ligament, inferiorly by the

urogenital diaphragm, anteriorly by the posterior wall of the bladder or posterior border of the external iliac vessel, posteriorly by the mesorectal fascia and uterosacral ligaments, and laterally by the pelvic sidewall. Specific details regarding the extent of parametria and vagina to be included in the CTV are outlined in more detail in the guidelines. A 1.5- to 2-cm primary/cervical CTV to PTV margin and a 7-mm nodal CTV to PTV margin are recommended. More generous margins should be used if only bone matching is used given the uncertainty of the primary CTV in relation to the nodal CTV. Daily imaging, discussed below, should be used to help prevent geographical target miss.

Given how recently these guidelines were published, there are no studies with long-term follow-up that have specifically used these guidelines. Multiple groups have, however, published their experiences with IMRT for definitive cervix treatment. One of the largest reports to date includes 81 patients that were treated using a 15-mm planning margin around the cervix, a 10-mm margin around the uterus, and a 7-mm margin around the remainder of the CTV (2). For stages I–IIA patients, the 3-year overall and disease-free survival rates were 77 and 70% compared with 62 and 51%, respectively, for stages IIB–IVA. Patients treated with cisplatin-based chemotherapy appeared to have lower acute and late toxicity compared with women treated in non-IMRT studies. Longer follow-up, more patients, and randomization are needed to solidify IMRT as a standard treatment option for definitive cervix treatment.

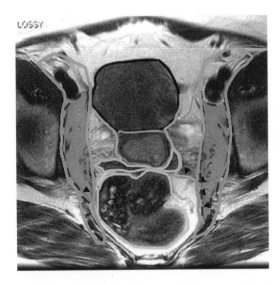

FIGURE 2 Consensus contours of the CTV and normal rectum on an MRI for the treatment of intact cervical carcinoma with IMRT.

■ IMAGE-GUIDED PTV MARGINS FOR EXTERNAL BEAM RADIATION THERAPY

The PTV margin accounts for target motion and patient set-up error. Trying to characterize target motion in gynecologic malignancies is complicated because it involves multiple mobile structures that can all move relative to one another and can be affected by bladder and rectal filling. The following section will review relevant literature that has characterized target motion in the postoperative and intact cervix settings as well as discuss the limitations of this information in creating generalized CTV to PTV margins.

Postoperative Cervix

Multiple studies have evaluated vaginal apex motion in the postoperative setting. One study followed up 22 women treated with postoperative pelvic IMRT with helical tomotherapy (23). To quantify the extent of vaginal wall organ motion, fiducial markers were placed in the vaginal apex prior to simulation. Marker position was measured on daily megavoltage (MV) computed tomography (CT) scans and compared with the index position on the initial planning CT scan. The authors noted the largest extent of motion was 12.1 mm in the anterior–posterior axis compared with only 3.1 mm in the right–left axis. Overall, 95% of all movements fell within 15.7 mm of their original position suggesting that, in most cases, a PTV margin of 16 mm would account for maximal organ motion.

In an another study, 24 patients status post hysterectomy received postoperative IMRT and had changes in the position of vaginal markers during the course of their treatment evaluated (24). Rescanning was performed twice weekly during IMRT. For the 16 women who had their vaginal markers in place throughout the course of IMRT, the median movement of the markers was 5.9 mm in the right–left direction, 14.6 mm in the anterior–posterior direction, and 12 mm in the superior–inferior direction. Also, despite specific bladder-filling instructions, there was considerable variability in bladder filling throughout the course of treatment. The median difference between the maximum and minimum bladder volumes was 247 cc (range, 96–585 cc). Large variations in bladder or rectal volume were also frequently correlated with significant vaginal apex displacement. These results emphasize that consistent bladder filling throughout the course of treatment is difficult to achieve and that solely relying on fiducial markers placed in the vaginal apex can be problematic as the markers may fall out.

In an another study, 14 patients (12 uterine cancer and 2 cervical cancer) status post hysterectomy were treated with postoperative radiation therapy (RT) and underwent MRI prior to starting treatment followed by weekly MRI scans during treatment (25). Similar to the above studies, the largest magnitude of CTV motion was in the anterior–posterior direction. A weak correlation in rectal filling and vaginal motion in the anterior–posterior direction and no correlation with bowel or bladder volumes were noted. With a homogenous CTV to PTV margin of

1.5 cm, ≥5% inadequate CTV coverage was only seen in 3.3% of cases.

The RTOG guidelines recommend using an internal target volume (ITV) approach to account for vaginal/parametrial motion. The CTV is defined on two CT scans obtained with a full as well as an empty bladder. These volumes should then be merged to create an ITV that accounts for movement of the vagina in relation to variations in daily bladder filling (9). No consensus PTV margin is recommend in the RTOG guidelines; however, a 1.0- to 1.5-cm (or institution-specific) uniform CTV expansion has been commonly advocated.

Intact Cervix

Determining "ideal" CTV to PTV margins in the intact cervix setting is more involved than in the postoperative setting. The uterus and the cervix are mobile structures that have variable movement, cervical tumors regress over time, and organ filling is a significant factor on CTV positioning.

Various imaging modalities and methods have been used to quantify motion in the intact cervical setting. One of the easiest and most widely available techniques is the use of portal imaging. One study, for example, looked at changes in the uterine sleeve position on portal films relative to the midline of the pubic symphysis in 3D. The investigators found that a PTV margin of 15.4, 17.5, and 22.9 mm in the superior–inferior, lateral, and anterior–posterior directions, respectively, would adequately dose the cervix in 95% of cases (14). Another study obtained anterior–posterior and lateral X-rays using on-board imaging (OBI) in 10 cervical cancer patients being treated with external beam RT to evaluate cervical marker seed motion (26). Interfraction movement in the lateral, vertical and anterior–posterior directions was 1.9 mm, 4.1 mm, and 4.2 mm with a range of 0 to 18 mm for each direction (SD ± 1.9, 2.4, and 2.7, respectively). The mean intrafraction movement in the lateral, vertical, and anterior–posterior directions was 1.6, 2.6, and 2.9 mm with a range of 1 to 15 mm for each direction (SD ± 2.0, 2.4, and 2.7, respectively). Overall, within and between radiation treatments, cervical motion averaged about 3 mm in any given direction, but the maximal movement could be as large as 18 mm from baseline.

Other groups have used CT scans to evaluate target motion over the course of treatment. A study of

13 cervical cancer patients treated with a small bowel displacement system had a CT scan for planning and then three weekly CT scans over the course of radiation (27). The position of the uterus was compared between the initial scan and subsequent ones. The most prominent interfraction change was in the superior–inferior direction. Also, even though there were relatively small interfraction position changes in the uterus with the use of the small bowel displacement system, there were large interpatient deviations.

MRI has also been used to investigate target motion in patients with intact cervical cancer. Thirty-three patients had changes in the position of the uterus and cervix assessed on MRI scans performed on 2 consecutive days during external beam RT (28). T2-weighted axial images were coregistered and the uterus and cervix were outlined on each scan. Three points (anterior uterine body, posterior cervix, and upper vagina) were identified and the displacement of each point was measured. They found that the movement of the uterus and the cervix was most pronounced in the superior–inferior and anterior–posterior directions. There was also greater movement noted in the uterus compared with the cervix. For example, the mean difference in anterior–posterior displacement between the uterus and the cervix was 7 versus 2.7 mm and in the superior–inferior direction was 7.1 versus 4.1 mm. The authors also found a correlation between bladder-filling and the superior-inferior movement of the uterus, whereas the anterior–posterior movement of the cervix and vagina was primarily affected by rectal filling. Based on these data, the recommendation is for an asymmetrical CTV to PTV expansion of the uterus: cervix and upper vagina of 15 mm anterior–posterior, 15 mm superior–inferior, and 7 mm laterally, and expansion of the nodal regions and parametria by 7 mm in all directions. Others have also observed that inter- and intrafraction motion is greatest at the fundus, less at the isthmus, and least at the cervical os (16).

In a different study, MRI scans obtained at the start of treatment and weekly during the first 4 weeks of chemoradiation were used to derive PTV margins on 20 patients (15). The investigators found that PTV margins of 24, 17, 12, 16, 11, and 8 mm in the anterior, posterior, right lateral, left lateral, superior, and inferior directions were needed to adequately cover the CTV. In this study, there was only a weak correlation between rectal volume changes and anterior–posterior CTV shifts.

Others have used cone beam computed tomography (CBCT) to evaluate target motion. In a study performed at the University of California San Diego (UCSD), kilovoltage (kV) CBCT was used to investigate the magnitude and impact of interfraction motion on CTV coverage in 10 patients (29). A CBCT was performed for each fraction and rigidly registered to the planning CT with respect to bony anatomy. The CTV from the planning CT was then cast onto each registered CBCT and modified by a radiation oncologist to adjust for changes due to organ motion and deformation thereby generating a new CTV for each fraction. The authors found that a uniform margin of 15 mm would have failed to encompass the entire CTV in 32% of the fractions and would have failed to encompass the cervix and fundus in 19 and 22% of the fractions, respectively. However, it needs to be noted that a 15-mm margin would on average have encompassed 99% of the CTV volume (range, 95–100%), and the average volume missed was 4 cc (range, 0–21 cc).

Aside from movement of the uterus and the cervix between fractions, consideration must also be given to tumor regression. Based on clinical examination, Lee and coworkers evaluated changes in tumor size for 17 cervical cancer patients during the course of definitive chemoradiation (14). High-dose rate brachytherapy was performed weekly starting about 2 to 3 weeks after the initiation of external beam RT. The average time for 50% tumor regression was 21 days and occurred after 30.8 Gy. Using weekly CT scans on 16 cervical cancer patients, investigators at the MD Anderson Cancer Center reported that there was a 62% mean volume reduction in the cervix after 45 Gy (30). Similarly, in a study of 14 patients with cervical cancer who underwent MR imaging before treatment and once during treatment, a 46% decrease in the primary gross tumor (range, 6–100%) was seen after approximately 30 Gy (31).

Another factor that is important to consider when constructing a PTV is bladder and rectal filling. The importance of this was shown in a study of 29 women with either cervical or endometrial cancer who had two planning CT scans. One scan was performed with an empty bladder and rectum and the other with a full bladder and rectum (12). Patients were treated in the prone position and the bladder and rectum were filled to a maximum extent with a mixture of 0.9% NaCl and contrast. The authors found the uterus moved, on average, 7 mm in the superior–inferior direction and 4 mm in the anterior–posterior direction depending on bladder and rectal filling. Rectal and bladder filling is not only important with respect to the position of the uterus and cervix, but also in regard to the dose the small bowel receives (32).

In summary, these studies show that there can be large inter- and intrafractional changes in the position of the uterus and cervix. These changes are only partially related to variations in bladder and/or rectal filling. For any given patient, these changes are not predictable or in the present day manageable and so it is critical when using IMRT to perform daily image guidance to verify that the CTV to PTV margin is adequately covering the target and not overdosing normal tissues.

■ IMAGE-GUIDED TARGET DELINEATION FOR BRACHYTHERAPY

The current standard of care for cervical cancer brachytherapy is to prescribe dose to Point A as defined by the International Commission on Radiation Units and Measurements (ICRU) using 2D imaging (33). Standard rectal and bladder dose constraints are also defined using points based on 2D imaging. With advances in 3D imaging, this 2D point system has been shown to not reliably cover the tumor, represent the maximum dose to OAR, or correlate well with acute or long-term toxicity (34,35). Consequently, significant work has gone into developing ways to define prescription doses and OAR dose constraints to volumes as opposed to points. The most extensive work in this area comes from using T2-weighted contrast-enhanced MRI to define specific target volumes. This sequence allows better differentiation of tumors from normal tissues and more accurate assessment of parametrial and uterine extension (36,37).

Given the improved soft tissue delineation with MRI, the Group Europeen de Curietherapie-European Society for Therapeutic Radiology and Oncology (GEC-ESTRO) and the North American Image-Guided Brachytherapy (IGBT) Working Group have published recommendations for MR-guided brachytherapy to help standardize and evaluate image-based dosimetry for cervical cancer brachytherapy (38–40). However, the nomenclature that has been adopted worldwide for IGBT is primarily based on the work performed by GEC-ESTRO (39,40).

Current recommendations for IGBT are to contour the GTV, the high-risk CTV (HR-CTV),

the intermediate-risk CTV (IR-CTV), and OARs including bladder, and rectum. The HR-CTV should include the entire cervix as well as any macroscopic disease that persists in the parametria, uterus, rectum, bladder, or vagina (but not to cross these anatomic boundaries without clear rationale). The prescription goal is 80 to 95 Gy to the HR-CTV. The IR-CTV should include tumor extension at diagnosis or a 1-cm extension around the HR-CTV, with the intent to deliver 60 Gy to this volume.

Recommendations for reporting and quality assurance (QA) include calculation and reporting of the minimum dose to 90 and 100% of the contoured target volume (D_{90}, D_{100}). In addition, for each implant, the volume encompassed by the 100% isodose line (V_{100}) should be calculated. The V_{150} and V_{200} should be calculated to determine volumes of tissue exceeding the prescription dose. For OARs, reporting of the ICRU reference points to the bladder and the rectum should continue for comparison with the dose-volume histogram (DVH) data. The minimum dose received by the maximally irradiated contiguous 0.1, 1, and 2 cm^3 of the bladder, rectum, and sigmoid should also be calculated and reported. Dose should be expressed as bioequivalent doses given at 2 Gy per fraction, using the linear quadratic radiobiologic model (EQD_2) to standardize for different dose rates (e.g., low-dose rate [LDR], HDR, and pulse-dose rate [PDR]). An excel spreadsheet template to help convert doses to EQD_2 is available online from the American Brachytherapy Society (ABS) website. Total doses should be expressed including the dose from external beam radiation. Provisional dose-volume constraints for OARs (converted to EQD_2) are to maintain the bladder below 85 to 90 Gy and the rectum and sigmoid below 75 Gy.

The largest experience implementing these recommendations has been carried out on a cohort of about 130 cervical cancer patients that have now been followed up for a median of 51 months (41). The use of IGBT compared with conventional brachytherapy resulted in improved local control in tumors >5 cm (64 vs. 82%, $p = .09$) and decreased late grade 3 and 4 GI and urinary morbidity (10 vs. 2%). The importance of dose to the HR-CTV in regard to local control was also demonstrated as patients with a D_{90} (EQD_2) ≥ 87 Gy had a >95% local control compared with only 80% for those with a D_{90} < 87 Gy (42). This was most pronounced for patients with >5 cm of residual disease at the time of brachytherapy. A recent publication on the validity of the OARs dosimetric constraints has also been reported (43). The authors found that a D_{2cc} rectal dose of 78 Gy results in a 10% probability of a grade ≥ 2 side effect. The dose for a 5% incidence of grade ≥ 2 side effect is in the range of 60 to 80 Gy. For the bladder, a D_{2cc} of 100 Gy corresponds to a 10% probability of a grade ≥ 2 side effect. The dose for a 5% probability ranges from 60 to 70 Gy.

Despite the advantages of MR-based planning, a 2007 survey found that the majority of radiation oncologists still use CT or planar imaging for brachytherapy planning (44). Underutilization of MR may be attributable in part to the lack of availability of MR-compatible applicators and/or onsite MR units. Given the availability of CT scanners in virtually all radiation oncology departments, a study was conducted comparing differences in GEC-ESTRO defined contours on CT versus MR images (45). Contouring on CT resulted in significantly wider HR-CTV and IR-CTV volumes compared with MR-based target contouring. The differences in width can significantly change the D_{90} and D_{100} and so MRI remains the standard for CTV delineation. Of note, the tumor height, thickness, total volume measurements, and OARs were similar between CT and MR based contouring. For clinics that are unable to obtain an MRI for brachytherapy planning, this paper provides guidelines for CT-based contouring of the HR-CTV and IR-CTV.

Another study comparing MRI with CT volumes demonstrated that while height, thickness, and especially width differed, the dosimetric differences were not so great as to preclude using one MRI but subsequently relying on CT's for planning (76).

Overall, despite the promising results of IGBT, its general adoption has been slow. The collaborative European study on MRI-guided brachytherapy in locally advanced cervical cancer (EMBRACE) will help provide important prospective evidence on the validation of the GEC-ESTRO recommendations in a multicenter setting.

■ IMAGE-GUIDED TREATMENT DELIVERY

To manage the regression and inter- and intrafractional movement of the cervix, image guidance during daily treatment may help ensure proper treatment delivery. Studies have shown that accurate positioning in gynecologic patients is difficult even when sophisticated customized immobilization and setup techniques are used (8,46). In fact, there is a wide range of opinions regarding the "ideal" way to simulate a patient. One study investigated the impact of patient positioning on PTV coverage in definitive cervical cancer treatment comparing patients in the prone position with and without a belly board as well as in the supine position (47). The authors found that the lowest risk of missing the PTV was when patients were in the prone position without a belly board. However, this needs to be balanced with other data that suggest belly boards can decrease dose to the small bowel in patients being treated for gynecologic cancers (46). There are other issues separate from patient positioning that also need to be accounted for in creating a reproducible set-up. Even greater difficulties may exist in setting up obese women and in patients treated with more comprehensive volumes, including extended-field RT and pelvic-inguinal RT. In-room IGRT approaches have the potential to improve set-up accuracy, reducing the risk of underdosing the target and overdosing nearby normal tissues. Another important problem that is addressed with in-room IGRT is accounting for internal organ motion, which can be dramatic for any one given patient.

■ CLINICAL APPLICATIONS OF IN-ROOM IGRT TECHNOLOGIES

There are currently no standard protocols for in-room IGRT in regard to the technique, frequency, or thresholds for replanning. In fact, while most radiation oncologists utilize IGRT for gynecologic patients, it is not a uniform practice. In a survey of radiation oncologists in the United States, 58% of respondents reported having used in-room IGRT in a patient with a gynecologic malignancy (48). The majority reported using planar-based techniques, particularly electronic portal imaging devices (EPIDs; 28%) and commercial OBI systems (24%). The percentage of respondents using volumetric-based techniques was also common, with 19% using kV and/or MV CBCT and 12% using helical tomotherapy. To date, no randomized trials have been reported to suggest that one form of daily imaging is superior or inferior to another. The type of imaging modality used is typically dictated by the available technology in that clinic.

EPID is the oldest and most commonly used IGRT modality (48). EPID uses the treatment beam or an X-ray imager mounted on the gantry to generate a 2D X-ray image. This image is then compared with a digitally reconstructed radiograph (DRR) from the planning CT scan, to make sure that there are no differences in the patient's positioning. An advantage of using EPID is that most modern linear accelerators are equipped with this technology; however, disadvantages include the time involved in obtaining frequent images during treatment and the potentially suboptimal quality of images obtained.

Multiple groups have used EPID in gynecologic patients to evaluate treatment set-up accuracy. One study of 14 patients undergoing pelvic irradiation used EPID to verify patient set-up and found that 57% of 254 fractions had set-up errors larger than 4 mm (11). In an another study, a prospective group of 20 women with gynecologic malignancies was divided into two groups. They were imaged and treated either on a conventional linear accelerator (LINAC) with planar kV and portal MV imaging or treated using helical tomotherapy with MV CT imaging (49). Errors in patient positioning ranged from 13 to 38 mm for patients imaged on the LINAC and 13 to 48 mm for those imaged with MV CT. Yamamoto and colleagues investigated the feasibility of delivering 3D conformal boosts using real-time tumor-tracking (RTRT) (50,51). These investigators used four sets of diagnostic X-ray tubes and imagers to monitor in real time the location of implanted cervical fiducial markers. The beam was "gated" to irradiate when the position of the markers coincided with their planned position. Using the RTRT system, the authors concluded that the CTV to PTV margin could be reduced to <1 cm in all directions. With a median follow-up of 17.6 months, complete response was achieved in nine patients and one had a partial response (50). The 2-year actuarial local-failure-free survival was 54% and the 2-year distant metastasis free survival was 72%. Late grade 2 rectal hemorrhage was seen in one patient.

Other radiation guidance techniques have been developed, which can generate 3D X-ray images. Commercially available examples include the ExacTrac system (BrainLAB, Feldkirchen, Germany) and CyberKnife (Accuray Inc., Sunnyvale, CA). These platforms utilize imaging systems that are mounted in the room to obtain high-resolution X-ray images that can be used for efficient and accurate target localization. One study compared intra- and interfraction motion in gynecologic patients receiving radiation using ExacTrac to conventional laser positioning and found no significant differences between the accuracy in positioning between the two systems (52). Investigators at the Korea Institute of Radiological and Medical Sciences reported outcomes on 30 patients with cervical or endometrial cancer with isolated paraaortic recurrences treated with a hypofractionated approach (33 to 34 Gy in three fractions) using the CyberKnife system (53). Gold fiducial markers were used to mark the tumor location and a custom-made device to limit respiratory motion was used at the time of simulation and during treatment. The PTV was defined as the GTV plus 2 mm. The 4-year actuarial overall survival rate was 50% and toxicity was low. These results are encouraging and demonstrate that high doses of radiation can be delivered, even to structures in the abdomen, effectively and with minimal toxicity.

Another method of IGRT utilizes soft-tissue imaging with CT scanning, with images acquired via either kV or MV systems. IGRT systems utilizing kV CT technology can be delivered in two ways. One is a conventional CT scanner that can be placed in the treatment room ("CT-on-rails"). This IGRT modality delivers the highest quality CT images, but lengthens treatment time, and cannot be used to detect intrafraction motion. A second approach is to install a kV X-ray source and detector directly onto the linear accelerator gantry. With a single 360 degree rotation of the gantry, daily kV CBCT images can be obtained. kV CBCT imaging systems have become an integrated option on most commercially available linear accelerator and provide another option for daily localization. At UCSD, daily image guidance using the OBI system was evaluated on a series of 10 gynecologic patients. The average shifts observed were 0.03 cm (range, –0.7 cm to 0.8 cm), –0.14 cm (range, –0.9 cm to 0.5 cm), and 0.08 cm (range, –0.5 cm to 0.5 cm) in the anterior–posterior, left–right, and superior–inferior directions, respectively (29).

Several vendors have developed gantry-mounted systems, using either the MV treatment beam itself or kV images generated by gantry-mounted sources to generate volumetric-based IGRT approaches. IGRT utilizing MV CT imaging can be performed in two ways. First, the EPID available on a conventional LINAC can be used to create an MV CBCT image. This method suffers from the limitation that patients are exposed to substantially higher doses of radiation outside the target because of the poor detection efficiency of X-ray detectors in the MV energy range. The second method of MV CT IGRT is helical tomotherapy (Hi-Art, Tomotherapy Inc.,

Madison, WI). This is an integrated imaging and treatment machine that combines a 6-MV energy LINAC with a diagnostic helical CT scanner. MV CT images are acquired immediately prior to treatment and aligned with the planning CT to verify the patient's position. Then, in a method similar to a diagnostic CT scan, the patient is treated in slices by a narrow photon beam that is modulated by binary multileaf collimators as the couch moves through the machine. Reports using helical tomotherapy and the Elekta kV CBCT (Elekta AB, Stockholm, Sweden) systems on gynecologic patients have been published showing sufficient image quality to perform set-up corrections (49,54).

There are multiple platforms available to carry out daily image guidance and whether one is better or worse than another is not known. The approach at UCSD with cervical cancer patients is that they are treated on a protocol using both planar and volumetric imaging with the OBI system. After the patient is aligned via skin marks, planar images are obtained with couch realignment performed remotely for all errors >1 mm. The patients then undergo a volumetric kV CBCT, the results of which are reviewed in real time and are used to ensure tumor coverage, although table movements based on the CT are rare as moving the field based on the primary tumor may compromise coverage of the nodal targets. If the target is felt to be inadequately covered it is most likely because of bladder or rectal filling and the patient is taken off the machine for correction and then treatment resumed. Luckily this is uncommonly necessary. An alternative approach under investigation is generation of several plans with real time selection based on the daily anatomy (55).

Aside from using modern imaging modalities to augment target delineation, IGRT also includes efforts to incorporate functional and/or biological information to help guide treatment planning. Incorporating functional or biological information into radiation treatment delivery has been investigated mostly in the setting of the definitive treatment of cervical cancer. For instance, investigators at Washington University have conducted several studies on PET-guided intracavitary brachytherapy (56–58). The procedure involves scanning patients after both intravenous delivery of ^{18}F-fluorodeoxyglucose (^{18}F-FDG) and insertion of tubes containing ^{18}F-FDG into the tandem and colpostats. The PET image is then transferred to the 3D planning system where volumes are delineated. In 11 cervical cancer patients a comparison was made between a standard brachytherapy plan designed to deliver 6.5 Gy to Point A with plans designed to conform to the 6.5 Gy isodose surface of a PET-defined volume. Although no difference was observed in target coverage for the first insertion, target coverage was significantly improved during later insertions using PET-based adaptive plans. There was, however, no difference observed in normal tissue sparing with the adaptive plans. Long-term outcomes using this approach are awaited. Other investigators have looked at PET with alternative tracers, such as ^{11}C-choline, ^{11}C-methinonine, and ^{60}Cu diacetyl-bis(N4-methylthiosemicarbazone) to identify metabolic abnormalities or hypoxia (59–62). The use of sophisticated imaging approaches to guide target delineation in gynecologic cancer patients is used at many centers (63).

Separate from target delineation, changes in PET standard uptake value (SUV) during the course of radiation may be able to be used to alter the course of treatment. A study by Schwarz and coworkers evaluated 36 cervical cancer patients with serial ^{18}F-FDG PET imaging before, during, and following chemoradiotherapy to see if changes in SUV were predictive (64). The mean maximum SUV observed at baseline, early treatment, midtreatment, late treatment, and posttreatment were 11.2 (range, 2.1–38), 5.5 (range, 0–25.2), 2.4 (range, 0–5.2), and 0.5 (range, 0–8.3), respectively. There was no correlation between treatment response and local or distant recurrence or survival. However, the overall data set was small and the timing of the PET scans varied considerably. Further work is needed to assess whether a subset of patients at high risk for recurrence could be identified by the metabolic response during treatment.

Aside from PET, MRI is increasingly used in radiation treatment planning. It has several advantages over CT-based planning, including increased soft tissue resolution and no radiation exposure to the patient. With MRI it is possible to contour a GTV and to follow changes in this volume over the treatment course. Investigators at Washington University performed weekly T2-fat saturated MRI scans for brachytherapy planning on 23 cervical cancer patients treated with definitive chemoradiotherapy (65). They found that a 30% drop in signal intensity from pretreatment to midtreatment correlated with disease resolution on posttreatment PET scan and with improved disease free survival compared to those who did not. Investigators at the Ohio State University followed up a group of 80 women with cervical cancer who had four MRI scans (before RT, during RT at 2–2.5 weeks, at 4–5 weeks, and 1–2 months after RT) for a median of 6.2 years (66). They found that both tumor volume and regression ratio were strongly correlated with local recurrence. The strongest predictor for local recurrence and tumor sterilization was the pre-RT volume and the regression ratio at 4 to 5 weeks during treatment.

MRI also has the ability to provide functional information by incorporating dynamic contrast enhancement (DCE) and diffusion-weighted imaging (DWI) sequences. The Ohio State University group has evaluated changes in DCE-MR over the course of treatment and its impact on clinical outcomes (67). Ninety-eight cervical cancer patients treated with chemoradiotherapy who had DCE-MRI performed before RT, during early RT (20–25 Gy), and mid-RT (45–50 Gy) were followed for a median of 4.9 years. Patients with an initial pre-RT high DCE had 100% 5-year local control, 81% disease-specific survival, and 81% overall survival compared with only 79, 61, and 55%, respectively, in patients with pre-RT low DCE. The authors hypothesized that the DCE levels reflect tissue oxygenation status and may serve as a potential noninvasive monitor of intratreatment radio-responsiveness that might be used to guide more personalized therapy.

With respect to DWI, less extensive work has been done, but one study of 15 patients with locally advanced cervical cancer performed an MRI that included T2-weighted and DWI sequences before the first and second fraction of brachytherapy (68). Apparent diffusion coefficients (ADC) were calculated and ADC maps were constructed and fused with GEC-ESTRO based contours. The mean ADC value within the GTV was significantly lower than in the HR-CTV which was also significantly lower than in the IR-CTV. There was no significant difference in the ADC values between the two brachytherapy insertions. This data validate the concept that the HR-CTV and IR-CTV have different quantities of residual disease at the time of brachytherapy; however, further studies are needed to evaluate the role of DWI in target contouring and dose prescription for image-guided brachytherapy.

While both PET and MRI provide valuable information that may be predictive and/or prognostic, it is not clear whether one of these modalities is superior to another. In fact, PET and MRI don't always encompass the same volume and so great care must be taken when basing contours on just a single imaging modality. This was demonstrated in a study in which 47 cervical cancer patients had both a PET/CT and MRI and the MRI-defined GTV was compared with the metabolic GTV as defined by PET/CT (65). The investigators noted significant discrepancies between the MRI GTV and the metabolic GTV, especially for tumors smaller than 14 cc.

While most IGRT efforts focus on defining and accurately targeting the CTV and PTV, image guidance can also be used to better define normal tissues. Early work by Roeske et al. found that single-photon emission CT (SPECT) could be used to image active bone marrow so that it could be selectively avoided during IMRT (69). Others have used [18F] FLT scans to identify active bone marrow regions to target as avoidance regions (70). While another group combined 18F-FDG PET with quantitative MR fat fraction maps to image structural and functional properties of the bone marrow to design bone-marrow-sparing IMRT plans (71). Whether efforts to limit active bone marrow versus more generalized constraints to the entire osseous pelvis are clinically meaningful is an active area of research.

■ FUTURE DIRECTIONS

While inter- and intra-fractional motions in the postoperative and intact cervix settings have been better characterized and quantified in recent years, further research is needed to explore how to best manage these motions. One possibility is to adapt plans during the course of treatment. Van de Bunt et al. investigated the impact of replanning cervical cancer patients undergoing definitive irradiation after 30 Gy based on repeat MRI (31). It was found that replanning significantly improved rectal sparing for all patients. The average rectal volume receiving 95% or more of the prescription dose was 75 cc (range, 20–145 cc) without replanning versus 67 cc (range, 15–106 cc) with replanning (p = .009). Small bowel sparing was also improved in women with bulky (>30 cc) tumors.

While this study demonstrates the feasibility of replanning and the potential benefit in dose to OARs it also raises some concerns. Given the significant inter-fractional changes in OARs and the target it is not clear whether adapting a plan midway through treatment will be optimal for subsequent treatments. It is even possible that an ideal plan on one day may actually be suboptimal on another. An example on how replanning may not always be optimal was shown by Lawson et al. who studied 10 cervical cancer patients receiving IMRT to assess the impact of midtreatment replanning using daily CBCT imaging (72). Replanning significantly improved CTV coverage with significant reductions seen in the small bowel and bladder. However, benefit in rectal sparing was mixed and in three patients, rectal irradiation was increased using the adapted plan.

Other groups have looked into the impact of weekly replanning. In one study, 11 cervical cancer patients had weekly MRI scans performed and four IMRT plans were created per patient to simulate an online-IMRT approach (73). Primary and nodal PTV margins were 15 and 10 mm for the pretreatment MRI scan but reduced to 4 mm for replanning. They contoured the bladder, rectum, bowel, sigmoid and looked at the dose distribution at six dose levels (V_{10}, V_{20}, V_{30}, V_{40}, $V_{42.8}$, and V_{45}). Online-IMRT compared with pre-IMRT significantly reduced the volume of normal tissue irradiated to all dose levels except V_{10}.

Apart from *whether* adaptation should be done, another question is *how* it should be done. One approach involves developing high-speed computing techniques for online treatment planning and optimization. The UCSD Center for Advanced Radiotherapy Technologies, in collaboration with researchers from the Lawrence Livermore Laboratories and the San Diego Supercomputer Center, has initiated a project known as SCORE (Super-Computing On-Line Re-planning Environment). The goal of the project is to allow image reconstruction, segmentation, deformation, replanning, and QA to be performed while the patient is on the treatment table (i.e., online). Recently, UCSD researchers have shown the feasibility of ultrafast IMRT plan optimization and dose calculation to facilitate online replanning (74,75).

An alternative approach is to develop a "library" of treatment plans before treatment. As envisioned, CBCT images would be obtained during treatment and used to select the most appropriate plan from the library. This plan would then be used to deliver treatment. Known as POLAR (Pre-planned On-Line Adaptive Radiotherapy), this approach is appealing, because all plans could undergo QA evaluation prior to their use. Multiple questions, however, remain regarding how many plans would be needed, how plans should be generated, and how the selection process should be accomplished. A concern with applying the POLAR approach to patients with cervical cancer is that a large library may be required, because of the degree of interfraction target motion caused by daily changes in rectal and bladder volumes.

■ CONCLUSIONS

Some general themes emerge from our current knowledge of IGRT for women with gynecologic malignancies. The first is that there are significant changes in both the target as well as the OARs throughout the course of treatment. Creating a standard CTV to PTV expansion for all patients will be appropriate for most women, but will miss outliers who have increased organ motion and tumor changes. It will also not capitalize on the goal of IGRT, which is to precisely deliver high doses of radiation to the target while minimizing dose to normal tissues. Approaches that individualize treatment margins are more likely to improve the therapeutic ratio of RT. Future directions that investigate either patient specific ITVs based on bladder filling and using daily imaging to pick a plan of the day versus online replanning using supercomputers are promising areas of research. Incorporation of functional imaging modalities, such as PET and MRI, are also likely to help individualize treatment. We have made significant progress in gynecologic IGRT and hopefully these advances will ultimately lead to improved treatment outcomes for these patients.

■ REFERENCES

1. Mell LK, Mehrotra AK, Mundt AJ. Intensity-modulated radiation therapy use in the U.S., 2004. *Cancer.* 2005;104:1296–1303.

2. Hasselle MD, Rose BS, Kochanski JD, et al. Clinical outcomes of intensity-modulated pelvic radiation therapy for carcinoma of the cervix. *Int J Radiat Oncol Biol Phys.* 2011;80:1436–1445.

3. Roeske JC, Lujan A, Rotmensch J, et al. Intensity-modulated whole pelvic radiation therapy in patients with gynecologic malignancies. *Int J Radiat Oncol Biol Phys.* 2000;48:1613–1621.

4. Mundt AJ, Lujan AE, Rotmensch J, et al. Intensity-modulated whole pelvic radiotherapy in women with gynecologic malignancies. *Int J Radiat Oncol Biol Phys.* 2002;52:1330–1337.

5. Mundt AJ, Mell LK, Roeske JC, et al. Preliminary analysis of chronic gastrointestinal toxicity in gynecology patients treated with intensity-modulated whole pelvic radiation therapy. *Int J Radiat Oncol Biol.* 2003;56:1354–1360.

6. Lujan AE, Mundt AJ, Roeske JC, et al. Intensity-modulated radiotherapy as a means of reducing dose to bone marrow in gynecologic patients receiving whole pelvic radiotherapy. *Int J Radiat Oncol Biol Phys.* 2003;57:516–521.

7. Mell LK, Tiryaki H, Ahn RH, et al. Dosimetric comparison of bone marrow-sparing intensity-modulated radiotherapy versus conventional techniques for treatment of cervical cancer. *Int J Radiat Oncol Biol Phys.* 2008;71:1504–1510.

8. Haslam JJ, Lujan AE, Mundt AJ, et al. Setup errors in patients treated with intensity-modulated whole pelvic radiation therapy for gynecological malignancies. *Med Dosim.* 2005;30:36–42.

9. Small W Jr., Mell LK, Anderson P, et al. Consensus guidelines for delineation of clinical target volume for intensity-modulated pelvic radiotherapy in postoperative treatment of endometrial and cervical cancer. *Int J Radiat Oncol Biol Phys.* 2008;71:428–434.

10. Lim K, Small W Jr., Portelance L, et al. Consensus guidelines for delineation of clinical target volume for intensity-modulated pelvic radiotherapy for the definitive treatment of cervix cancer. *Int J Radiat Oncol Biol Phys.* 2011;79:348–355.

11. Stroom JC, Olofsen-van Acht MJJ, Quint S, et al. On-line set-up corrections during radiotherapy of patients with gynecologic tumors. *Int J Radiat Oncol Biol Phys.* 2000;46:499–506.

12. Buchali A, Koswig S, Dinges S, et al. Impact of the filling status of the bladder and rectum on their integral dose distribution and the movement of the uterus in the treatment planning of gynaecological cancer. *Radiother Oncol.* 1999;52:29–34.

13. Huh, SJ, Park W, Han Y. Interfractional variation in position of the uterus during radical radiotherapy for cervical cancer. *Radiother Oncol.* 2004;71:73–79.

14. Lee CM, Shrieve DC, Gaffney DK. Rapid involution and mobility of carcinoma of the cervix. *Int J Radiat Oncol Biol Phys.* 2004;58:625–630.

15. van de Bunt L, Jürgenliemk-Schulz IM, de Kort GA, et al. Motion and deformation of the target volumes during IMRT for cervical cancer: What margins do we need? *Radiother Oncol.* 2008;88:233–240.

16. Chan P, Dinniwell R, Haider MA, et al. Inter- and intra-fractional tumor and organ movement in patients with cervical cancer undergoing radiotherapy: A cinematic-MRI point-of-interest study. *Int J Radiat Oncol Biol Phys.* 2008;70:1507–1515.

17. Taylor A, Powell MEB, Quint S, et al. An assessment of interfractional uterine and cervical motion: Implications for radiotherapy target volume definition in gynaecological cancer. *Radiother Oncol.* 2008;88:250–257.

18. Vilarino-Varela MJ, Taylor A, Rockall AG, et al. A verification study of proposed pelvic lymph node localisation guidelines using nanoparticle-enhanced magnetic resonance imaging. *Radiother Oncol.* 2008;89:192–196.

19. Jhingran A, Portelance L, Winter K, et al. Phase II study of pelvic intensity modulated radiotherapy +/- chemotherapy for post-operative patients with endometrial or cervical carcinoma (RTOG 0418) [abstract]. *Int J Radiat Oncol Biol Phys.* 2010;75:1034.

20. Portelance L, Chao KSC, Grigsby PW, et al. Intensity-modulated radiation therapy (IMRT) reduces small bowel, rectum, and bladder doses in patients with cervical cancer receiving pelvic and para-aortic irradiation. *Int J Radiat Oncol Biol Phys.* 2001;51:261–266.

21. Gerszten K, Colonello K, Heron DE, et al. Feasibility of concurrent cisplatin and extended field radiation therapy (EFRT) using intensity-modulated radiotherapy (IMRT) for carcinoma of the cervix. *Gynecol Oncol.* 2006;102:182–188.

22. Beriwal S, Gan GN, Heron DE, et al. Early clinical outcome with concurrent chemotherapy and extended-field, intensity-modulated radiotherapy for cervical cancer. *Int J Radiat Oncol Biol Phys.* 2007;68:166–171.

23. Harris EER, Latifi K, Rusthoven C, et al. Assessment of organ motion in postoperative endometrial and cervical cancer patients treated with intensity-modulated radiation therapy. *Int J Radiat Oncol Biol Phys.* 2011 (in press).

24. Jhingran A, Salehpour M, Sam M, et al. Vaginal motion and bladder and rectal volumes during pelvic intensity-modulated radiation therapy after hysterectomy. *Int J Radiat Oncol Biol Phys.* 2011 (in press).

25. Jürgenliemk-Schulz IM, Toet-Bosma MZ, de Kort GA, et al. Internal motion of the vagina after hysterectomy for gynaecological cancer. *Radiother Oncol.* 2011;98:244–248.

26. Haripotepornkul NH, Nath SK, Scanderbeg D, et al. Evaluation of intra- and inter-fraction movement of the cervix during intensity modulated radiation therapy. *Radiother Oncol.* 2011;98:347–351.

27. Lee JE, Han Y, Huh SJ, et al. Interfractional variation of uterine position during radical RT: Weekly CT evaluation. *Gynecol Oncol.* 2007;104:145–151.

28. Taylor A, Rockall AG, Reznek RH, et al. Mapping pelvic lymph nodes: Guidelines for delineation in intensity-modulated radiotherapy. *Int J Radiat Oncol Biol Phys.* 2005;63:1604–1612.

29. Tyagi N, Lewis JH, Yashar CM, et al. Daily online cone beam computed tomography to assess interfractional motion in patients with intact cervical cancer. *Int J Radiat Oncol Biol Phys.* 2011;80:273–280.

30. Beadle BM, Jhingran A, Salehpour M, et al. Cervix regression and motion during the course of external beam chemoradiation for cervical cancer. *Int J Radiat Oncol Biol Phys.* 2009;73:235–241.

31. van de Bunt L, van der Heide UA, Ketelaars M, et al. Conventional, conformal, and intensity-modulated radiation therapy treatment planning of external beam radiotherapy for cervical cancer: The impact of tumor regression. *Int J Radiat Oncol Biol Phys.* 2006;64:189–196.

32. Han Y, Shin EH, Huh SJ, et al. Interfractional dose variation during intensity-modulated radiation therapy for cervical cancer assessed by weekly CT evaluation. *Int J Radiat Oncol Biol Phys.* 2006;65:617–623.

33. International Commission on Radiation Units and Measurements: ICRU Report 38: *Dose and volume specification for reporting intracavitary therapy in gynecology.* Bethesda, MI.

34. Datta NR, Srivastava A, Maria Das KJ, et al. Comparative assessment of doses to tumor, rectum, and bladder as evaluated by orthogonal radiographs vs. computer enhanced computed tomography-based intracavitary brachytherapy in cervical cancer. *Brachytherapy.* 2005;5:223–229.

35. Kim RY, Shen S, Duan J. Image-based three-dimensional treatment planning of intracavitary brachytherapy for cancer of the cervix: Dose-volume histograms of the bladder, rectum, sigmoid colon, and small bowel. *Brachytherapy.* 2006;6:187–194.

36. Dimopoulos JCA, Schard G, Berger D, et al. Systematic evaluation of MRI findings in different stages of treatment of cervical cancer: Potential of MRI on delineation of target, pathoanatomic structures, and organs at risk. *Int J Radiat Oncol Biol Phys.* 2006;64:1380–1388.

37. Zwahlen D, Jezioranski J, Chan P, et al. Magnetic resonance imaging-guided intracavitary brachytherapy for cancer of the cervix. *Int J Radiat Oncol Biol Phys.* 2009;74:1157–1164.

38. Nag S, Cardenes H, Chang S, et al. Proposed guidelines for image-based intracavitary brachytherapy for cervical carcinoma: Report from Image-Guided Brachytherapy Working Group. *Int J Radiat Oncol Biol Phys.* 2004;60:1160–1172.

39. Haie-Meder C, Pötter R, Van Limbergen E, et al. Recommendations from Gynaecological (GYN) GEC-ESTRO Working Group[star, open] (I): concepts and terms in 3D image based 3D treatment planning in cervix cancer brachytherapy with emphasis on MRI assessment of GTV and CTV. *Radiother Oncol.* 2005;74:235–245.

40. Pötter R, Haie-Meder C, Kirisits C, et al. Recommendations from gynaecological (GYN) GEC ESTRO working group (II): Concepts and terms in 3D image-based treatment planning in cervix cancer brachytherapy—3D dose volume parameters and aspects of 3D image-based anatomy, radiation physics, radiobiology. *Radiother Oncol.* 2006;78:67–77.

41. Pötter R, Dimopoulos J, Georg P, et al. Clinical impact of MRI assisted dose volume adaptation and dose escalation in brachytherapy of locally advanced cervix cancer. *Radiother Oncol.* 2007;83:148–155.

42. Dimopoulos JCA, Pötter R, Long S, et al. Dose-effect relationship for local control of cervical cancer by magnetic resonance image-guided brachytherapy. *Radiother Oncol.* 2009;93:311–315.

43. Georg P, Pötter R, Georg D, et al. Dose effect relationship for late side effects of the rectum and urinary bladder in magnetic resonance image-guided adaptive cervix cancer brachytherapy. *Int J Radiat Oncol Biol Phys.* 2011 (in press).

44. Viswanathan AN, Erickson BA. Three-dimensional imaging in gynecologic brachytherapy: A survey of the American Brachytherapy Society. *Int J Radiat Oncol Biol Phys.* 2010;76:104–109.

45. Viswanathan AN, Dimopoulos J, Kirisitis C, et al. Computed tomography versus magnetic resonance imaging-based contouring in cervical cancer brachytherapy: Results of a prospective trial and preliminary guidelines for standardized contours. *Int J Radiat Oncol Biol Phys.* 2007;68:491–498.

46. Olofsen-van Acht M, van den Berg H, Quint S, et al. Reduction of irradiated small bowel volume and accurate patient positioning by use of a bellyboard device in pelvic radiotherapy of gynecological cancer patients. *Radiother Oncol.* 2001;59:87–93.

47. Weiss E, Eberlein K, Pradier O, et al. The impact of patient positioning on the adequate coverage of the uterus in the primary irradiation of cervical carcinoma: a prospective analysis using magnetic resonance imaging. *Radiother Oncol.* 2002;63:83–87.

48. Simpson DR, Lawson JD, Nath SK, et al. A survey of image-guided radiation therapy use in the United States. *Cancer.* 2010;116:3953–3960.

49. Santanam L, Esthappan J, Mutic S, et al. Estimation of setup uncertainty using planar and MVCT imaging for gynecologic malignancies. *Int J Radiat Oncol Biol Phys.* 2008;71:1511–1517.

50. Yamamoto RA, Yonesaka A, Nishioka S, et al. High dose three-dimensional conformal boost (3DCB) using an orthogonal diagnostic X-ray set-up for patients with gynecological malignancy: A new application of real-time tumor-tracking system. *Radiother Oncol.* 2004;73:219–222.

51. Park HC, Shimizu S, Yonesaka A, et al. High dose three-dimensional conformal boost using the real-time tumor tracking radiotherapy system in cervical cancer patients unable to receive intracavitary brachytherapy. *Yonsei Med J.* 2010;51:93–99.

52. Weiss E, Vorwerk H, Richter S, et al. Interfractional and intrafractional accuracy during radiotherapy of gynecologic carcinomas: A comprehensive evaluation using the ExacTrac system. *Int J Radiat Oncol Biol Phys.* 2003;56:69–79.

53. Choi CW, Cho CK, Yoo SK, et al. Image-guided stereotactic body radiation therapy in patients with isolated para-aortic lymph node metastases from uterine cervical and corpus cancer. *Int J Radiat Oncol Biol Phys.* 2009;74:147–153.

54. McBain CA, Henry AM, Syked J, et al. X-ray volumetric imaging in image-guided radiotherapy: The new standard in on-treatment imaging. *Int J Radiat Oncol Biol Phys.* 2006;64:625–634.

55. Yashar C, Cornell M, Mell L, et al. *Feasibility of dynamic adaptive radiotherapy for cervical carcinoma.* International Gynecologic Cancer Society, Prague, Czech Republic. October 23 2010.

56. Malyapa RS, Mutic S, Low DA, et al. Physiologic FDG-PET three-dimensional brachytherapy treatment planning for cervical cancer. *Int J Radiat Oncol Biol Phys.* 2002;54:1140–1146.

57. Mutic S, Grigsby PW, Low DA, et al. PET-guided three-dimensional treatment planning of intracavitary gynecologic implants. *Int J Radiat Oncol Biol Phys.* 2002;52:1104–1110.

58. Lin LL, Mutic S, LaForest R, et al. Adaptive brachytherapy treatment planning for cervical cancer using FDG-PET. *Int J Radiat Oncol Biol Phys.* 2007;67:91–96.

59. Lapela M, Leskinen-Kallio S, Varpula M, et al. Imaging of uterine carcinoma by carbon-11-methionine and PET. *J Nucl Med.* 1994;35:1618–1623.

60. Dehdashti F, Grigsby PW, Mintun MA, et al. Assessing tumor hypoxia in cervical cancer by positron emission tomography with 60Cu-ATSM: Relationship to therapeutic response—a preliminary report. *Int J Radiat Oncol Biol Phys.* 2003;55:1233–1238.

61. Torizuka TK, Kanno T, Futatsubashi M, et al. Imaging of gynecologic tumors: Comparison of (11)C-choline PET with (18)F-FDG PET. *J Nucl Med.* 2003;44:1051–1056.

62. Grigsby P, Malyapa RS, Higashikubo R, et al. Comparison of molecular markers of hypoxia and imaging with (60) Cu-ATSM in cancer of the uterine cervix. *Mol Imaging Biol.* 2007;9:278–283.

63. Simpson DR, Lawson JD, Nath SK, et al. Utilization of advanced imaging technologies for target delineation in radiation oncology. *J Am Coll Radiol.* 2009;6:876–883.

64. Schwarz JK, Lin LL, Siegel BA, et al. 18-F-fluorode-oxyglucose-positron emission tomography evaluation of early metabolic response during radiation therapy for cervical cancer. *Int J Radiat Oncol Biol Phys.* 2008;72:1502–1507.

65. Ma DJ, Zhu J-M, Grigsby PW. Tumor volume discrepancies between FDG-PET and MRI for cervical cancer. *Radiother Oncol.* 2011;98:139–142.

66. Wang JZ, Mayr NA, Zhang D, et al. Sequential magnetic resonance imaging of cervical cancer. *Cancer.* 2010;116:5093–5101.

67. Mayr N, Wang JZ, Zhang D, et al. Longitudinal changes in tumor perfusion pattern during the radiation therapy course and its clinical impact in cervical cancer. *Int J Radiat Oncol Biol Phys.* 2010;77:502–508.

68. Haack S, Pedersen EM, Jespersen SN, et al. Apparent diffusion coefficients in GEC ESTRO target volumes for image guided adaptive brachytherapy of locally advanced cervical cancer. *Acta Oncol.* 2010;49:978–983.

69. Roeske JC, Lujan A, Reba RC, et al. Incorporation of SPECT bone marrow imaging into intensity modulated whole-pelvic radiation therapy treatment planning for gynecologic malignancies. *Radiother Oncol.* 2005;77:11–17.

70. McGuire SM, Menda Y, Ponto LL, et al. A methodology for incorporating functional bone marrow sparing in IMRT planning for pelvic radiation therapy. *Radiother Oncol.* 2011;99:49–54.

71. Mell L, Liang Y, Bydder M, et al. Functional MRI-guided bone marrow-sparing intensity modulated radiotherapy for pelvic malignancies [abstract]. *Int J Radiat Oncol Biol Phys.* 2009;75:S121.

72. Lawson JD, Simpson DR, Roese BS, et al. Adaptive radiotherapy in cervical cancer: Dosimetric analysis using daily cone-beam CT [abstract]. *Int J Radiat Oncol Biol Phys.* 2009;75:S85–86.

73. Kerkhof EM, Raaymakers BW, van der Heide UA, et al. Online MRI guidance for healthy tissue sparing in patients with cervical cancer: An IMRT planning study. *Radiother Oncol.* 2008;88:241–249.

74. Gu X, Men C, Choi D, et al. GPU-based ultra-fast dose calculation using a finite size pencil beam model. *Phys Med Biol.* 2009;54:6287–6297.

75. Men C, Choi D, Majumdar A, et al. GPU-based ultrafast IMRT plan optimization. *Phys Med Biol.* 2009;54:6565–6573.

76. Eskander RN, Scanderbeg D, Saenz CC, et al. Comparison of computed tomography and magnetic resonance imaging in cervical cancer brachytherapy target and normal tissue contouring. *Int J Gynecol Cancer.* 2010; 20(1):47–53.

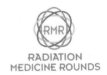

RADIATION
MEDICINE ROUNDS

Image-Guided Brachytherapy in Cervical Cancer

Akila N. Viswanathan*

*Department of Radiation Oncology, Brigham and Women's Hospital/
Dana-Farber Cancer Institute, Harvard Medical School, Boston, MA*

■ ABSTRACT

Compared with X-ray–based brachytherapy, the use of three-dimensional images for planning brachytherapy provides a much more precise estimation of dose to the tumor and to the surrounding normal tissues. The use of standardized guidelines over the past 5 years has created a common language for communication and research, resulting in a uniform format internationally to report outcome data, including local recurrence and toxicity results. Future improvements in individualizing patient treatments using more advanced imaging technologies potentially include refining the precision of targeting and permitting dose modulation based on the amount of residual disease present at the time of brachytherapy.

Keywords: cervical cancer, brachytherapy, image guidance, magnetic resonance imaging, computed tomography

■ INTRODUCTION

Cervical cancer is the most common gynecologic tumor worldwide, often afflicting young women in their ages 30s to 40s; appropriate diagnosis and treatment therefore result in significant benefits to society (1). Treatment for women with locally advanced cervical cancer requires concurrent chemotherapy with radical radiation including both external-beam radiation therapy (EBRT) and internal brachytherapy (2). Worldwide, the majority of institutions utilize plain films (Figure 1) for gynecologic brachytherapy planning, with radiation dose calculated at a point, rather than to a volume (3,4). Over the past 10 years, interest has surged in three-dimensional (3D)–based brachytherapy for assistance with insertion (via ultrasound [US]) and planning (via computed tomography [CT], magnetic resonance imaging [MRI] or positron-emission tomography [PET]). The result has been an appreciation of individual patient and tumor image-detected characteristics. 3D imaging of brachytherapy applicator placement, when used to aid treatment planning,

*Corresponding author, Brigham and Women's Hospital/
Dana-Farber Cancer Institute, Harvard Medical School, 75
Francis Street L2, Boston, MA 02115
 E-mail address: aviswanathan@lroc.harvard.edu

Radiation Medicine Rounds 2:3 (2011) 371–382.
DOI: 10.5003/2151-4208.2.3.371

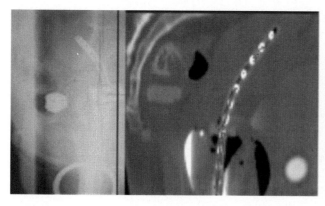 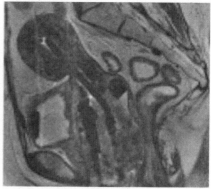

FIGURE 1 A comparison of plain film X-ray, CT, and 3-T MRI imaging for brachytherapy demonstrates the ability of plain films to show the applicator, but not soft tissue; the ability of CT to show the organs at risk (OAR) but not the tumor; and the ability of MRI to show the tumor and OAR.

increases the precision of radiation dose delivery by defining the tumor, resulting in maximum sparing of the normal tissues (5). Several institutions have explored the use of image-guided brachytherapy to conformally treat the tumor and avoid the normal tissues, with institutional data indicating an increase in survival and reduction in toxicity related to imaging during brachytherapy.

■ ROLE OF IMAGE-GUIDED BRACHYTHERAPY VERSUS AN EBRT BOOST

Despite the increased risks to the surrounding normal tissues and the lack of large trials supporting the use of additional EBRT as a sequential boost, highly conformal methods of EBRT, such as intensity-modulated radiation (IMRT) and stereotactic body radiation (SBRT), have been proposed as theoretical alternatives to image-guided brachytherapy after initial EBRT. However, studies to date using external beam as an alternative boost instead of brachytherapy demonstrate significantly inferior survival rates compared with those that use brachytherapy. One argument has been to use external beam as a boost for patients that cannot undergo tandem placement (Figure 2). However, the use of US to guide the insertion enables tandem placement in almost all cases, even when the os cannot be identified. In one study from Manchester, United Kingdom, 44 patients with cervical cancer who could not receive brachytherapy for various reasons (6) instead received EBRT to 54 to 70 Gy via a 3D conformal boost in most cases. After a median follow-up of 2.3 years, 48% relapsed with 16

of 21 developing a central recurrence. The 5-year overall survival rate was 49%, significantly lower than for a comparable brachytherapy-treated group. A treatment planning report compared inversely planned EBRT with photons (IMRT) and protons to 3D MRI-guided brachytherapy (7). EBRT was programmed to deliver the highest possible doses to the planning target volume (PTV), while respecting D_{2cc} limits from brachytherapy, assuming the same fractionation. Volumes receiving 60 Gy (in equivalent dose in 2-Gy fractions) were approximately twice as large for IMRT compared with brachytherapy, and the high-central tumor dose was lower than that seen with brachytherapy. This led the authors to conclude that for cervix-cancer boost treatments, both IMRT and protons are inferior to 3D-image–based brachytherapy.

Two inherent problems with IMRT or SBRT exist: the need for continual replanning given rapid tumor regression and internal organ motion (8–10), and the increase in integral dose, with normal tissues throughout the pelvis receiving more radiation than with brachytherapy. In one study, mean maximum changes in the center of the cervix were 2.1, 1.6, and 0.82 cm in the superior–inferior, anterior–posterior, and right–left lateral dimensions, respectively (11). Another study identified that within and between radiation treatments, cervical motion averaged approximately 3mm in any given direction with maximal movement of the cervix up to 18mm from baseline. Given the large movement, and the increased dose to the normal tissues resulting in an increase in normal-tissue toxicity, highly conformal (IMRT, SBRT) methods for boosting the cervix are not recommended (12,13). All of the OAR move significantly between fractions, necessitating

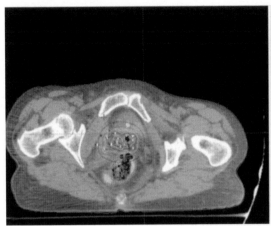 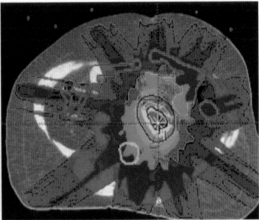

FIGURE 2 A comparison of the dose distribution between brachytherapy (left image) and IMRT (right) showing that IMRT results in a significantly higher integral dose and can produce excessive bowel dose given the significant bowel movement over a course of treatment, whereas the brachytherapy applicator moves with the center of the tumor.

replanning for accurate OAR dose assessment. (move reference 24 Holloway et al. to #14)

■ DOSE RATE AND GENERAL RADIOBIOLOGIC PRINCIPLES

For brachytherapy, the International Commission on Radiation Units and Measurements (ICRU) in its Report 38 (15) defines ranges of brachytherapy dose rate as: low dose rate (LDR), 0.4 to 2 Gy/hr; medium dose rate (MDR), 2 to 12 Gy/hr; and high dose rate (HDR), over 12 Gy/hr. Though image guidance may be used for any dose rate, the greatest benefit is seen when the modality allows the greatest flexibility with dose optimization. Given the stepping source computer-optimized planning in HDR and pulsed-dose-rate (PDR) brachytherapy, one may maximize tumor dose and minimize the normal-tissue damage that can occur with large fraction sizes with these systems. The linear-quadratic (LQ) model allows calculation of an estimated biologically equivalent dose adjusted for dose rate, dose per fraction, and overall treatment time (16,17). For comparison, the LQ model doses are normalized to an equivalent dose in 2 Gy (EQD2) (18). The LQ model, relying on the α/β ratio, estimates and compares equivalent doses for various time-dose-fractionation schemes (19). For cervical cancer, an α/β ratio of 10 Gy is used for tumor and 3 Gy for normal tissues (20), which may be an underestimate for a squamous cell carcinoma and an overestimate for the rectum (21), though an α/β ratio of 3 Gy for the rectum has

been correlated with late rectal complications (22,23). Spreadsheets to assist with dose calculations can be found at www.americanbrachytherapy.org/guidelines.

■ IMAGING MODALITIES USED IN IMAGE-GUIDED BRACHYTHERAPY

Ultrasound

Of all of the available 3D imaging methods, US has several advantages. It is quick, accessible, cost-effective, lacks ionizing radiation, and is the most commonly available 3D imaging modality for brachytherapy procedures worldwide. 3D US transducers may depict tumor volume measurements that are generally considered more accurate than conventional 2D thickness measurements. Doppler US shows dynamic vascular flow information via either color flow, which detects blood flow direction and velocity, or power mode Doppler, which improves sensitivity for flow detection, but does not provide information regarding the flow direction or velocity. Regarding US probe configuration, transabdominal or transrectal probes are used in gynecologic brachytherapy. Transabdominal probes are typically used to assist with tandem insertion into the uterus, and may help identify interstitial catheters as inserted into the cervix. Transabdominal US can measure uterine width and height in patients who do not have large fibroids or tumor volumes that greatly distort uterine configuration. Transrectal US may be used for interstitial brachytherapy. It allows visualization of posterior interstitial catheters as they traverse the cervix and enter the uterus, but as the great majority of cases have an anteverted uterus, a transrectal probe cannot be used to assist with tandem insertion. Therefore, if only one probe is available, a transabdominal probe is preferred. US assessment of the brachytherapy applicator in situ is a safe and reliable method to confirm applicator position midline in the myometrium. In the United States, US is primarily used to aid with applicator insertion (24). To date, only one Australian group has compared cervical cancer dimensions obtained with US to those obtained with MRI to aid with brachytherapy planning. US was found to be comparable with MRI for defining target volume and rectal point, though dose-volumetric information for the organs at risk (OAR) was not available (25). US images may not have as clear a resolution as CT or MRI, though methods to determine the utility of US to assist with treatment planning are of interest for future research.

Computed Tomography

With the installation of CT simulators in Radiation Oncology clinics in the United States, more physicians have integrated CT imaging into their brachytherapy practice. For gynecologic brachytherapy, a CT is most commonly performed after insertion in a separate procedure room. The CT images confirm that a perforation did not occur during the insertion. The images may also be used for treatment planning, to contour 3D volumes of the OAR (bladder, rectum, and sigmoid) and the uterine cervix. However, despite having a CT scanner, most clinics continue to use point dosimetry for treatment planning. Optimization of dose away from the normal tissues is best achieved by placing contrast into the organs before a CT, then optimizing the dose away from these regions while covering the tumor. In LDR brachytherapy, there is less ability to optimize the dose distribution, as one is limited by the available Cesium strength.

CT represents a significant contribution over radiographic X-ray film, with its point-based dosimetry, for OAR dose estimation. It also provides a reasonable estimation of the location of the cervix. The CT contours of the cervix overestimate the tumor contours compared with an MRI, though the additional width contoured on a CT may be of benefit to the patient, as cervical cancer tends to spread laterally along the parametrial tissues. However,

radiation-related changes in the parametria, uterus, and cervix may not be reliably estimated on CT.

Due to lack of tissue contrast (Figure 1), CT does not clearly delineate tumor tissue from the adjacent uterus, parametrial tissue, or other normal tissue. Though CT images may be used for OAR contouring and dose-volume-histogram (DVH) analysis, it may not provide sufficient detail of the tumor to allow dose conformality to the tumor and away from the normal tissues when compared with MRI (26–28). The uterus and cervix appear homogeneous on a CT, and the only distinction between these two structures may be made by inference regarding their size and location. Gross residual disease in the cervix cannot be distinguished from the myometrium or adjacent involved parametrium.

CT can relay information to the observer about changes in the OAR related to tumor shrinkage, organ motion, and the location of the brachytherapy applicator in relation to the uterus. OAR contour accuracy may be increased by placing contrast into the bladder and rectum. Optimization of the OAR based on CT is similar to that based on MRI. Loops of bowel adjacent to the uterus or cervix may have the same enhancement and distinguishing this interface on CT may be difficult. A slice thickness of 2.5 mm is often used for applicator assessment. Intravenous (IV) contrast is difficult to properly time during brachytherapy and therefore is not recommended; its utility is simply to identify the uterine arteries, which help delineate the superior border of the cervix. Rectal contrast is often administered to aid with contouring of the rectal wall. Bladder contrast may be utilized for patients receiving brachytherapy who have a Foley catheter in place.

In a recent multicenter study jointly conducted by the American College of Radiology Imaging Network (ACRIN) and the Gynecologic Oncology Group (GOG), MRI was significantly better than CT for tumor visualization and detection of parametrial involvement (28). CT typically overestimates the tumor width, but may be used in gynecologic brachytherapy with good results if MRI is not available. Though MRI more accurately defines a tumor volume, whether it confers a significant clinically relevant benefit compared with CT has not been tested in a clinical trial.

Magnetic Resonance Imaging

MRI offers several advantages over other imaging modalities, including its inherent multiplanar capability, lack of ionizing radiation, and excellent soft-tissue contrast resolution. MRI can provide highly accurate assessment of the extent of local tumor invasion of other pelvic structures such as the parametria, vagina, bladder, and rectum. The strength of a magnet in an MR scanner is expressed by a unit of measurement called Tesla (T). The higher the field strength, the better the overall signal-to-noise ratio (SNR), resulting in more accurate imaging.

MRI using T1- and/or T2-weighted images has been reported to be superior to any other available modality in imaging the normal anatomy of the female pelvis. Fluid is dark on T1-weighted images, whereas fluid is bright on T2-weighted images. Cancer is better depicted on T2-weighted images, due to the presence of edema. For cervical cancer, multiplanar axial, sagittal, and coronal, T2-weighted, fast spin-echo images with a small field of view are performed. Registration and fusion of MR and CT images may increase the clarity, given potential image distortion with high T MR images and the lack of contrast in the cervix on CT. For diagnostic scans, vaginal contrast with US gel may improve visualization of the vaginal walls and lower parts of the cervix. For brachytherapy, MRI-compatible applicators, vaginal packing impregnated with and a Foley catheter filled with contrast medium leads to clear visualization of relevant structures. Bowel motion can be reduced by intravenous or intramuscular drug administration.

Over the course of EBRT, radiation-induced changes may be detected by MR and this may predict clinical outcomes, including local recurrence and survival. In a prospective study performed by Mayr et al., 34 patients with cervical cancer of various stages underwent 1.5 T MRI before and after radiation therapy. Tumor volumetry (3D measurements) was obtained using T2-weighted images to quantify the tumor regression rate. Sequential tumor volumetry using MRI was found to be a very effective measure of the responsiveness of cervical cancer to irradiation (29).

Given the shrinkage of the tumor and changes in the OAR between brachytherapy fractions, accurate target and organ delineation is critical for optimizing the treatment to permit dose escalation to the target while sparing the OAR. Careful analysis of cross-sectional images with particular attention to tumor regression and regions of potential tumor spread is critical. T2-weighted, fast recovery, fast spin-echo MR images with 1-mm isotropic voxel size oriented parallel and orthogonal to the applicator (sources) axes permit imaging in the plane of the brachytherapy applicator (30).

Positron Emission Tomography

PET-CT using fluorodeoxyglucose (FDG) contrast has been shown to be very effective for the staging of cervical cancer. Dosimetric studies with PET in brachytherapy demonstrate interesting results (31), but to date no clinical trials with PET in brachytherapy have been published. PET-CT provides highly accurate localization of focal radiotracer uptake, which significantly improves the diagnostic accuracy compared with PET or CT alone. Most cervical squamous cell carcinomas are FDG avid. FDG uptake is commonly seen in the adjacent vagina, uterus, bladder or parametrial region in the setting of localized tumor extension. Normal physiologic FDG excretion into the urinary bladder may result in false-positive involvement. Complete bladder voiding prior to imaging is essential.

Contouring and Dosimetric Nomenclature

Traditionally, the dose from the brachytherapy applicator was specified at point A, identified on an anterior pelvic radiograph with the applicator in place. Point A has been used systematically for cervical cancer dose specification since the 1930s, and is defined as a point 2 cm from the tandem, and 2 cm superior to the upper surface of the vaginal applicator. In the era of HDR brachytherapy, where the room for error is much greater given the high dose per fraction, rapid dose fall off, brief treatment time, and narrowing of the therapeutic ratio, proper applicator placement and precise estimation of the location of the normal tissues are of key importance. With imaging, one may visualize the tumor volume and dose-adapt to either reduce the dose to point A (covering a smaller tumor volume) or escalate the dose to point A (covering a large tumor volume extending beyond the boundaries of point A) (Figure 3). In the modern era, with the widespread availability of 3D imaging, point-based radiographic dosimetry has limited utility for the dose adaptation required when using HDR brachytherapy. Point A may overestimate or underestimate the tumor dose as determined on 3D imaging (32). The tumor coverage always depends on tumor volume at the time of brachytherapy, with

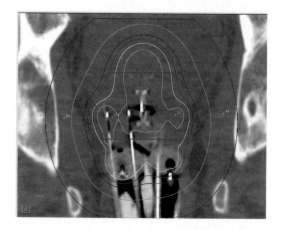

FIGURE 3 After EBRT, CT images used for brachytherapy treatment planning may show how the traditional point A lies inside or outside of the cervix, and would over- or under-treat the region. Some cases have a large amount of residual disease (image) and require moving the 100% isodose line beyond point A. In this case, a combination of tandem and ovoids with needles was used to dose escalate the large volume of residual disease.

larger tumors less likely to be encompassed by the prescribed isodose (32–34). However, it is recommended to report the dose to point A to ensure consistency in terminology and reporting between centers (26).

The importance of the clinical gynecologic examination cannot be underestimated in gynecologic brachytherapy (35,36). Clinical evaluation of the extent of disease at the time of diagnosis, remission during EBRT, and residual tumor at the time of brachytherapy may indicate the extent of vaginal involvement, the lateral and anterior–posterior dimensions of the tumor, and any suspicious rectal-wall invasion. Placing radio-opaque marker seeds at the time of diagnosis marking the inferior, lateral, and superior extensions of a vaginal tumor is very helpful for identifying regions requiring dose escalation with brachytherapy. The clinical findings should be documented by schematic drawings of tumor extension initially and at the time of brachytherapy and these should be made available for appropriate target volume delineation and dose estimation. Selecting the proper applicator (tandem/ring, tandem/ovoid, tandem/interstitial, or tandem/cylinder) is paramount to ensure adequate coverage of the disease.

Combined with the clinical examination, sectional imaging provides a way to view and delineate the tumor and OAR. Errors in contouring of either the target or the OAR reduce the potential accuracy of treatment. Due to inhomogeneous dose distributions and sharp dose fall-off, even minimal delineation inaccuracies can dramatically change dosing to normal-tissue structures. Therefore, formal education programs with contouring are paramount to increasing interobserver agreement (30).

In 2005, both the American Brachytherapy Society and the Groupe Europeen Curietherapy-European Society for Therapeutic Radiation Oncology (GEC-ESTRO) agreed to incorporate guidelines (35,36) into future studies utilizing MR-based planning. The recommended delineated volumes on MRI include a gross tumor volume (GTV), including all T2-bright areas of enhancement. The high-risk clinical target volume (HR-CTV) includes the entire cervix as well as any regions of high to intermediate signal intensity in the parametria, uterus, or vagina, and any residual disease detected on clinical examination at the time of brachytherapy. The intermediate-risk clinical target volume (IR-CTV) includes the tumor extension at the time of diagnosis, and adds 1 cm to the HR-CTV volume, subtracting out the OARs. The IR-CTV represents areas harboring potential microscopic metastatic disease in the regions surrounding the areas where gross disease was present.

For CT-scanned cases when MR is not available (37), an HR-CTV can be contoured based on the lateral borders of the cervix and any parametrial extension detected. Uterosacral ligaments may be visualized on CT and, if detected, they should be included in the HR-CTV contours. Whether the overestimation required with CT contouring due to the lack of clarity of the exact tumor volume is of benefit in terms of providing extra dose to the potential tumor-containing regions, or if this may be more detrimental than the more precise MR volumes, has not been conclusively determined.

With the GEC-ESTRO recommendations, the primary dose-volume parameters reported for target structures (HR-CTV) are D_{90}, D_{100}, and V_{100}. D_{90}, defined as the dose received by at least 90% of the target volume, is most commonly used for reporting and comparing dose values. The cumulative D_{90} equals the sum of D_{90}s from the individual fractions plus the dose from a homogeneous 3D conformal external-beam treatment (38,39). D_{100}, the minimum target dose, may be more sensitive to inaccuracies in contouring and dose calculation. The V_{100}

assesses dose coverage of the whole target volume, and is 100% when the entire target is covered by the prescribed dose. V_{150} and V_{200} are often reported in interstitial brachytherapy. Prescribed dose is based on the physician's directive of the dose intended for the target volume. During treatment planning, dose optimization techniques attempt to cover the target volume to the prescribed dose.

The OAR, including the bladder, rectum and sigmoid, may be contoured on any 3D modality. With CT or MRI, contrast placed into the OAR assists with identification. However, contrast may cause some artifact, resulting in some variation in contouring the wall of the organ. The OAR can be contoured by outlining either the whole organ with its contents or the organ wall. When outlining the whole organ, the regions of highest delineated dose may not be located entirely within the organ wall, if the wall is very thin. Wachter-Gerstner et al. analyzed the correlation between dose-volume histograms (DVHs) for bladder and rectum, based on whole-organ and organ-wall volumes. The D_{2cc} served as a good estimate for doses to the organ wall, whereas the D_{5cc} was dependent on filling status (40). Olzsewska et al. showed that rectal wall thickness did not significantly impact the D_{2cc} value (41).

For the OAR, ICRU 38 point doses have been traditionally used. Recently, several studies found that the ICRU bladder point may underestimate maximum doses (42,43); it is less likely that ICRU rectal doses will incorrectly estimate the maximum dose. A sigmoid dose is not calculated in the ICRU system given the difficulty with identifying the sigmoid. Numerous publications do support a correlation between the ICRU point dose and the probability of late complications for bladder and rectum (44,45).

DVH analysis correlates doses with volumes rather than points; and DVH metrics may provide a reliable predictor of long-term complications (46). The dose to the OAR is reported by cumulative DVH parameters, including the D_{2cc} and $D_{0.1cc}$. The D_{2cc} is the minimum dose received by the most exposed 2 cm^3 volume of the analyzed organ. Georg et al. recently tested the predictive value of dose-volume parameters for late effects of the rectum, sigmoid, and bladder using the D_{2cc}, D_{1cc}, and $D_{0.1cc}$ of these three OARs for 141 cervical cancer patients treated with 3D EBRT and MRI-guided brachytherapy. The mean D_{2cc} values for bladder, rectum, and sigmoid were 95 ± 22 Gy, 65 ± 12 Gy, and 62 ± 12

Gy, respectively. This study confirmed that D_{2cc} was a predictor of late toxicity for the rectum and bladder (46).

Koom et al. showed that patients with a higher D_{2cc} had significantly more severe rectal side effects (endoscopy score ≥2) (47). Seventy-one patients with FIGO Stage IB–IIIB uterine cervical cancer underwent CT-based HDR intracavitary brachytherapy. The mean values of the DVH parameters and ICRU rectal point were significantly greater in patients with a score of >2 than in those with a score <2 at 12 months after brachytherapy (ICRU α/β = 3, 71 vs. 66 Gy, p = .02; $D_{0.1cc}$, 93 vs. 85 Gy, p = .04; D_{1cc}, 80 vs. 73 Gy, p = .02; D_{2cc}, 75 vs. 69 Gy, p = .02). The probability of a score of >2 was significantly correlated with the DVH parameters and ICRU rectal point (ICRU, p = .03; $D_{0.1cc}$, p = .05; D_{1cc}, p = .02; D_{2cc}, p = .02).

In Vienna, a rectoscopy study was done in 35 patients (48), in which the total doses were normalized to 2-Gy fractions (EQD2, α/β = 3 Gy), in 0.1, 1.0, and 2.0 cm^3 ($D_{0.1cc}$, D_{1cc}, D_{2cc}) of rectum. After a mean follow-up time of 18 months, telangiectasia was found in 26 patients (74%), five had ulceration corresponding to the 0.1 cm^3 volume (anterior wall). Mean values for $D_{0.1cc}$, D_{1cc}, and D_{2cc} were 81 ± 13, 70 ± 9, and 66 ± 8 Gy, respectively. D_{2cc} was higher in patients with rectoscopy score ≥3 compared with <3 (72 ± 6 vs. 62 ± 7 Gy; p < .001) and in symptomatic versus asymptomatic patients (72 ± 6 vs. 63 ± 8 Gy; p < .001). The localization of these changes corresponds to the high-dose volumes as defined by imaging. The development of mucosal and clinical changes in the rectum seems to follow a clear dose effect and volume effect. Based on these two studies, we recommend a dose limit of 70 to 75 Gy EQD2 for the rectal dose constraint.

Timing and Recommended Doses

Tumor regression during EBRT is about 70 to 80% of the pretherapeutic tumor volume (27–30). All treatment should be completed within 8 weeks (31–33). Therefore, brachytherapy should start between weeks 4 to 5 of EBRT. There is no advantage to starting the brachytherapy early as the goal is to shrink the tumor as much as possible prior to brachytherapy to maximize a reproducible and ideal geometry of the applicator. If the applicator is placed in the presence of significant tumor (week 2), the geometry will change dramatically, reducing the ability to minimize OAR dose.

For cervical cancer in the United States, the most common EBRT dose treats the elective pelvic nodes to 45 to 50 Gy given in 1.8 Gy/fraction (24). For HDR, in the United States, typically five fractions are administered (5–6 Gy per fraction), with two fractions per week. Brachytherapy follows, with a goal EQD2 dose of 80 to 90 Gy to the HR-CTV (24–26). One study found that a dose to the HR-CTV over 87 Gy resulted in a local recurrence rate of 4% compared with 20% for a D_{90} < 87 Gy when the tumor was >5 cm and using an HDR tandem/ring or tandem/ring/interstitial approach. They concluded that local control rates >95% can be achieved for patients with a poor response after EBRT if the D_{90} for the HR-CTV is 87 Gy or higher. The IR-CTV intended dose should be about 60 Gy EQD2.

DVH constraints for both PDR (17,19–21) and HDR (18,43) are 90 Gy (EQD2) for bladder and 70 to 75 Gy (EQD2) for both rectum and sigmoid as minimal doses to the most exposed 2 cm³ of the OAR. The clinical relevance of using a 70- to 75-Gy constraint for rectum has recently been demonstrated (52). There are no generally accepted constraints for the 0.1-cm³ level. Given the rapid regression of the tumor, and the dramatic change in the location and size of the normal tissues, it is recommended to replan and determine the doses to the OAR with each fraction.

■ CLINICAL OUTCOMES

Applicator: Tandem and Ring/Tandem and Ovoid/Mould

At the present time, several centers are accruing cases of MRI-guided brachytherapy for cervical cancer to the European registry EMBRACE. Single institutions have previously reported their experience to date. The Medical University of Vienna, using a 0.2-T MRI, has reported their clinical outcomes for 145 patients with Stage IB–IVA cervical cancer treated with 4 fractions of 7 Gy HDR from 1998 to 2003 (49). Complete remission was achieved in 138 patients (95%), with seven patients having locally persistent or progressive disease in the central (*n* = 5) or noncentral (*n* = 2) pelvis. With a median follow-up of 40 months, the 4-year local control rate was 83% compared with 63% for historical controls.

Investigators at the Institut Gustave Roussy (IGR) reported on 45 patients treated between 2004 and 2006 with a tandem and mould technique using PDR brachytherapy and MR-based contouring (50). Until recently at IGR, surgery was often performed after brachytherapy if disease was suspected on clinical examination. A dose of ≥15 Gy (after EBRT) was prescribed to the IR-CTV. The dose to the HR-CTV was about 250% of the dose to the IR-CTV (i.e., 80 Gy to the HR-CTV). With a median follow-up of 26 months, one local recurrence has occurred. Very recently, data on 39 patients treated at IGR with MRI-guided LDR brachytherapy in the preoperative setting was published (51). A total dose of 60 Gy to the IR-CTV was followed 6 weeks later by extrafascial hysterectomy and bilateral salpingo-oophorectomy with pelvic node dissection. Adjuvant chemoradiation was delivered to patients with pelvic lymph node involvement. After a median follow-up of 4.4 years (range, 2.6 to 6.6 years), there were no central recurrences; one local recurrence occurred in the lateral pelvis (2.6%). The 4-year actuarial overall and disease-free survival rates were 94 and 86%, respectively. The 2- and 4-year actuarial local relapse-free survival rates were 94 and 91%, respectively.

Two other European centers [34,52] and one Canadian center (53) have reported feasibility data for MR-based cervical-cancer brachytherapy, showing a reduction in the normal-tissue toxicity rate. These centers confirm that using 0.5 to 1.5 T MR-based tandem/ring or tandem/ovoid brachytherapy with MRI is feasible, and that outcome measures appear favorable. At Tata Memorial Hospital in India, 24 patients with squamous cell cervical carcinoma were treated with MRI-based HDR. With a median follow-up of 12 months (54), two patients had local failures (21).

CT-based therapy has been reported by a few institutions. The Addenbrooke Hospital reported on 28 patients with a median follow-up of 23 months after HDR 8 Gy × 3 CT-guided brachytherapy (55). The 3-year actuarial cancer-specific survival rate in this group was 81%, with a pelvic control rate of 96%. Five of the 28 patients died of paraaortic or other distant disease, one of them being the only one with local recurrence presenting as a malignant vesico-vaginal fistula. In 24 patients, a D_{90} ≥74 Gy was achieved. The only patient with local recurrence had a D_{90} of 63.8 Gy; this was a 20% improvement over historic non-image-guided controls.

Toxicities

In the Vienna series, the actuarial grade 3 to 4 late morbidity at 3 years were gastrointestinal 4%, urinary 4%, and vaginal 5%. Two patients required permanent colostomies for grade 4 complete obstruction of the recto-sigmoid junction. Two patients suffered from grade 3 persistent rectal bleeding and required blood transfusions. Two patients developed grade 4 severe late adverse effects in the urinary bladder 3 to 4 years after treatment, with refractory cystitis and excruciating dysuria, and consequently both underwent cystectomy (56). One patient experienced grade 3 urinary incontinence, with 1 to 2 h interval frequency, which started during treatment. The great majority of grade 1 to 2 late vaginal effects were asymptomatic; when symptomatic, patients presented with dryness and atrophy of the vaginal epithelium or partial synechiae and stenosis of the upper vagina. Five patients experienced grade 3 coaptation of the vagina.

At IGR, of the 45 patients studied, 23 and 2 patients developed acute grade 1 to 2 and grade 3 complications, respectively; 21 patients presented with delayed grade 1 to 2 complications. One other patient presented with a grade 3 vesicovaginal fistula. No grade 4 or greater complications, whether acute or delayed, were observed. In the IGR experience, a total of 20 grade 1 to 2 late complications were observed in 13 patients (33%): 10 urinary bladder, 3 ureteral, 1 rectal, 1 small bowel, 1 vaginal, 1 pelvic fibrosis, 1 peripheral nerve, and 2 others. No grade 3 or 4 complication occurred.

Tan et al. (55) reported on 28 patients treated with CT-guided brachytherapy for Stage IB-IIIB cervix cancer. Their overall actuarial 3-year grade 3 to 4 morbidity rate was 14%. Two patients had grade 3 abdominal pain and one had a colo-vaginal fistula. Overall, the data indicate that a potential reduction in morbidity appears to be a benefit of image-guided brachytherapy.

Applicator: Template-Based Interstitial

The first prospective trial of real-time MRI guidance during interstitial gynecologic therapy (57) treated 25 patients and recorded one sigmoid-vaginal fistula, where the vaginal-apex tumor was adherent to the sigmoid and regression of the tumor resulted in the opening of a previously unknown fistula tract

(58). A report on the use of tandem/short interstitial needles for cervical cancer described clinical outcomes in 22 patients followed for a median of 20 months; no grade 3 or 4 toxicities were noted, and one patient had a local recurrence (59). Dose optimization with either PDR or HDR may improve the normal-tissue doses for interstitial therapy for some patients.

The University of Pittsburgh reported on 11 cervical cancer patients treated with CT-guided HDR interstitial brachytherapy (5 fractions of 3.5 Gy per fraction) (60). From 1998 to 2004 interstitial brachytherapy was chosen for cases with distorted anatomy or extensive vaginal disease. The 5-year actuarial local control rate was 63%. No patient had acute grade 3 or 4 toxicity. Grade 3 or 4 late toxicity occurred in one patient with a 5-year actuarial rate of 7%. Three patients had late grade 2 rectal toxicity and one patient had grade 2 small-bowel toxicity.

Syed et al. reported an approximately 10% toxicity rate with long-term follow-up (61) without 3D planning. An approximate 11% rate of bowel insertion and a long-term fistula rate of 4 to 10% have been reported in studies using CT for planning after insertion (26,27).

■ CONCLUSION

3D image-guided brachytherapy for cervical cancer has increased dramatically over the past 10 years. Institutional studies indicate promising improvements in local control and survival. Future prospective clinical trials will provide more information enabling individualization of cervical cancer brachytherapy.

■ REFERENCES

1. WHO. *Age-Standardized Incidence Rates of Cervical Cancer. 2009.* [May 22, 2010]; Available from: http://www.who.int/mediacentre/factsheets/fs297/en/

2. Rose PG, Eifel, PJ. Combined modality treatment for carcinoma of the cervix. In: Hellman S, DeVita V, Rosenberg S, eds. *Principles and Practices of Oncology Updates.* New York, NY: Lippincott Williams and Wilkins, 2000:1–10.

3. Viswanathan AN, et al. International brachytherapy practice patterns: A survey of the Gynecologic Cancer Intergroup (GCIG). *Int J Radiat Oncol Biol Phys.* Epub 2010.

4. Viswanathan AN, Erickson BA, Three-dimensional imaging in gynecologic brachytherapy: A survey of the American Brachytherapy Society. *Int J Radiat Oncol Biol Phys.* 2010;76(1):104–109.

5. Viswanathan AN, et al. *Gynecologic Radiation Therapy: Novel Approaches to Image-Guidance and Management.* Berlin: Springer; 2011:308.

6. Barraclough LH, et al. External beam boost for cancer of the cervix uteri when intracavitary therapy cannot be performed. *Int J Radiat Oncol Biol Phys.* 2008;71(3):772–778.

7. Georg D, et al. Image-guided radiotherapy for cervix cancer: High-tech external beam therapy versus high-tech brachytherapy. *Int J Radiat Oncol Biol Phys.* 2008;71(4):1272–1278.

8. Lim K, et al. Cervical cancer regression measured using weekly magnetic resonance imaging during fractionated radiotherapy: Radiobiologic modeling and correlation with tumor hypoxia. *Int J Radiat Oncol Biol Phys.* 2008;70(1):126–133.

9. Lee CM, Shrieve DC, Gaffney DK. Rapid involution and mobility of carcinoma of the cervix. *Int J Radiat Oncol Biol Phys.* 2004;58(2):625–630.

10. van de Bunt L, et al. Motion and deformation of the target volumes during IMRT for cervical cancer: What margins do we need? *Radiother Oncol.* 2008;88(2):233–240.

11. Beadle BM, Jhingran A, Salehpour M, Sam M, Iyer RB, Eifel PJ. Cervix regression and motion during the course of external beam chemoradiation for cervical cancer. *Int J Radiat Oncol Biol Phys.* 2009;73:235–241.

12. Haripotepornkul NH, Nath SK, Scanderbeg D, Saenz C, Yashar CM. Evaluation of intra- and inter-fraction movement of the cervix during intensity modulated radiation therapy. *Radiother Oncol.* 2011;98:347–351.

13. Tyagi N, Lewis JH, Yashar CM, et al. Daily online cone beam computed tomography to assess interfractional motion in patients with intact cervical cancer. *Int J Radiat Oncol Biol Phys.* 2011;80:273–280.

14. Holloway C, et al. Sigmoid dose using 3D imaging in cervical cancer brachytherapy. *Radioth Oncol.* 2009;93(2):307–310.

15. ICRU 38, *Dose and volume specifications for reporting intracavitary therapy in gynecology*, 1985, International Commission on Radiation Units and Measurements: Bethesda MD. p. 1–23.

16. Dale RG, The application of the linear quadratic dose-effect equation to fractionated and protracted radiotherapy. *Br J Radiol.* 1985;58:515–528.

17. Joiner MC, van der Kogel AJ. The linear quadratic approach to fractionation and calculation of isoeffect relationships. In: Steel GG, ed. *Basic Clinical Radiobiology.* London: Arnold, 1997:106–122.

18. Lang S, et al. Intercomparison of treatment concepts for MR image assisted brachytherapy of cervical carcinoma based on GYN GEC-ESTRO recommendations. *Radiother Oncol.* 2006;78(2):185–193.

19. Bentzen SM, Joiner MC, The linear quadratic approach in clinical practice. In: Joiner MC, van der Kogel AJ, eds. *Basic Clinical Radiobiology.* London: Hodder Arnold, 2009:120–134.

20. Potter R, et al. Recommendations from gynaecological (GYN) GEC ESTRO working group (II): Concepts and terms in 3D image-based treatment planning in cervix cancer brachytherapy-3D dose volume parameters and aspects of 3D image-based anatomy, radiation physics, radiobiology. *Radiother Oncol.* 2006;78:67–77.

21. Sturdza A, Potter R. Outcomes related to the disease and the use of 3D-based external beam radiation and image-guided brachytherapy. In: Viswanathan AN, et al., eds. *Gynecologic Radiation Therapy: Novel Approaches to Image-Guidance and Management.* Berlin: Springer, 2011:263–282.

22. Noda SE, et al. Late rectal complications evaluated by computed tomography-based dose calculations in patients with cervical carcinoma undergoing high-dose-rate brachytherapy. *Int J Radiat Oncol Biol Phys.* 2007;69(1):118–124.

23. Clark BG, et al. The prediction of late rectal complications in patients treated with high dose rate brachytherapy for carcinoma of the cervix. *Int J Radiat Oncol Biol Phys.* 1997;38(5):989–993.

24. Watkins JM, et al. Ultrasound-guided tandem placement for low-dose-rate brachytherapy in advanced cervical cancer minimizes risk of intraoperative uterine perforation. *Ultrasound Obstet Gynecol.* 2011;37(2):241–244.

25. Van Dyk S, et al. Conformal brachytherapy planning for cervical cancer using transabdominal ultrasound. *Int J Radiat Oncol Biol Phys.* 2009;75(1):64–70.

26. Eisbruch A, et al. Customized gynecologic interstitial implants: CT-based planning, dose evaluation, and optimization aided by laparotomy. *Int J Radiat Oncol Biol Phys.* 1998;40(5):1087–1093.

27. Erickson B, Albano K, Gillin M. CT-guided interstitial implantation of gynecologic malignancies. *Int J Radiat Oncol Biol Phys.* 1996;36(3):699–709.

28. Hricak H, et al. Early invasive cervical cancer: CT and MR imaging in preoperative evaluation—ACRIN/GOG comparative study of diagnostic performance and interobserver variability. *Radiology.* 2007;245(2):491–498.

29. Mayr NA, et al. Tumor perfusion studies using fast magnetic resonance imaging technique in advanced cervical cancer: A new noninvasive predictive assay. *Int J Radiat Oncol Biol Phys.* 1996;36(3):623–633.

30. Petric P, et al. Inter- and intraobserver variation in HR-CTV contouring: intercomparison of transverse and paratransverse image orientation in 3D-MRI assisted cervix cancer brachytherapy. *Radiother Oncol.* 2008;89(2):164–171.

31. Lin LL, et al. Adaptive brachytherapy treatment planning for cervical cancer using FDG-PET. *Int J Radiat Oncol Biol Phys.* 2007;67(1):91–96.

32. Kim RY, Pareek P. Radiography-based treatment planning compared with computed tomography (CT)-based treatment planning for intracavitary brachytherapy in cancer of the cervix: analysis of dose-volume histograms. *Brachytherapy.* 2003;2(4):200–206.

33. Datta NR, et al. Comparative assessment of doses to tumor, rectum, and bladder as evaluated by orthogonal radiographs vs. computer enhanced computed tomography-based intracavitary brachytherapy in cervical cancer. *Brachytherapy.* 2006;5(4):223–229.

34. Lindegaard JC, et al. MRI-guided 3D optimization significantly improves DVH parameters of pulsed-dose-rate brachytherapy in locally advanced cervical cancer. *Int J Radiat Oncol Biol Phys.* 2008;71(3):756–764.

35. Haie-Meder C, Potter R, Van Limbergen E, et al. Recommendations from Gynaecological (GYN) GEC-ESTRO Working Group (I): Concepts and terms in 3D image based 3D treatment planning in cervix cancer brachytehrapy with emphasis on MRI assessment of GTV and CTV. *Radiother Oncol.* 2005;74:235–245.

36. Potter R, et al. Recommendations for image-based intracavitary brachytherapy of cervix cancer: The GYN GEC ESTRO Working Group point of view: In regard to Nag et al. (Int *J Radiat Oncol Biol Phys.* 2004;60:1160–1172). *Int J Radiat Oncol Biol Phys.* 2005;62(1):293–295; author reply 295–296.

37. Viswanathan AN, et al. Computed tomography versus magnetic resonance imaging-based contouring in cervical cancer brachytherapy: results of a prospective trial and preliminary guidelines for standardized contours. *Int J Radiat Oncol Biol Phys.* 2007;68(2):491–498.

38. Kirisits C, et al. Dose and volume parameters for MRI-based treatment planning in intracavitary brachytherapy for cervical cancer. *Int J Radiat Oncol Biol Phys.* 2005;62(3):901–911.

39. Chargari C, et al. Physics contributions and clinical outcome with 3D-MRI-based pulsed-dose-rate intracavitary brachytherapy in cervical cancer patients. *Int J Radiat Oncol Biol Phys.* 2009;74(1):133–139.

40. Wachter-Gerstner N, et al. Bladder and rectum dose defined from MRI based treatment planning for cervix cancer brachytherapy: comparison of dose-volume histograms for organ contours and organ wall, comparison with ICRU rectum and bladder reference point. *Radiother Oncol.* 2003;68(3):269–276.

41. Olszewska AM, et al. Comparison of dose-volume histograms and dose-wall histograms of the rectum of patients treated with intracavitary brachytherapy. *Radiother Oncol.* 2001;61(1):83–85.

42. Ling CC, et al. CT-assisted assessment of bladder and rectum dose in gynecological implants. *Int J Radiat Oncol Biol Phys.* 1987;13:1577–1582.

43. Schoeppel SL, et al. Three-dimensional treatment planning of intracavitary gynecologic implants: analysis of ten cases and implications for dose specification. *Int J Radiat Oncol Biol Phys.* 1994;28(1):277–283.

44. Kim HJ, et al. Are doses to ICRU reference points valuable for predicting late rectal and bladder morbidity after definitive radiotherapy in uterine cervix cancer? *Tumori.* 2008;94(3):327–332.

45. Chen SW, et al. Comparative study of reference points by dosimetric analyses for late complications after uniform external radiotherapy and high-dose-rate brachytherapy for cervical cancer. *Int J Radiat Oncol Biol Phys.* 2004;60(2):663–671.

46. Georg P, et al. Dose-volume histogram parameters and late side effects in magnetic resonance image-guided adaptive cervical cancer brachytherapy. *Int J Radiat Oncol Biol Phys.* 2011;79(2):356–362.

47. Koom WS, et al. Computed tomography-based high-dose-rate intracavitary brachytherapy for uterine cervical cancer: preliminary demonstration of correlation between dose-volume parameters and rectal mucosal changes observed by flexible sigmoidoscopy. 2007;68(5):1446–1454.

48. Georg P, et al. Correlation of dose-volume parameters, endoscopic and clinical rectal side effects in cervix cancer patients treated with definitive radiotherapy including MRI-based brachytherapy. 2009;91(2):173–180.

49. Potter R, et al. Clinical impact of MRI assisted dose volume adaptation and dose escalation in brachytherapy of locally advanced cervix cancer. *Radiother Oncol.* 2007;83(2):148–155.

50. Chargari C, et al. Physics contributions and clinical outcome with 3D-MRI-based pulsed-dose-rate intracavitary brachytherapy in cervical cancer patients. *Int J Radiat Oncol Biol Phys.* 2009;74(1):133–139.

51. Haie-Meder C. DVH parameters and outcome for patients with early-stage cervical cancer treated with preoperative MRI-based low dose rate brachytherapy followed by surgery. *Radiother Oncol.* 2009;93(2) L316–L321.

52. De Brabandere M, et al. Potential of dose optimisation in MRI-based PDR brachytherapy of cervix carcinoma. *Radiother Oncol.* 2008;88(2):217–226.

53. Zwahlen D, et al. Magnetic resonance imaging-guided intracavitary brachytherapy for cancer of the cervix. *Int J Radiat Oncol Biol Phys.* 2009;74(4):1157–1164.

54. Cozzi L, et al. A treatment planning study comparing volumetric arc modulation with RapidArc and fixed field IMRT for cervix uteri radiotherapy. *Radiother Oncol.* 2008;89(2):180–191.

55. Tan LT, et al. Clinical impact of computed tomography-based image-guided brachytherapy for cervix cancer using the tandem-ring applicator—the Addenbrooke's experience. *Clin Oncol. (R Coll Radiol)* 2009;21(3):175–182.

56. Potter R, et al. 3D conformal HDR-brachy- and external beam therapy plus simultaneous cisplatin for high-risk cervical cancer: Clinical experience with 3 year follow-up. *Radiother Oncol.*, 2006(0167–8140 (Print)).

57. Viswanathan AN, et al. Magnetic resonance-guided interstitial therapy for vaginal recurrence of endometrial cancer. *Int J Radiat Oncol Biol Phys.* 2006;66(1):91–99.

58. Viswanathan A, et al. Final results of a prospective study of MR-based interstitial gynecologic brachytherapy. *Brachytherapy.* 2008;7:148.

59. Dimopoulos JC, et al. The Vienna applicator for combined intracavitary and interstitial brachytherapy of cervical cancer: Clinical feasibility and preliminary results. *Int J Radiat Oncol Biol Phys.* 2006;66(1):83–90.

60. Beriwal S, et al. Early clinical outcome with concurrent chemotherapy and extended-field, intensity-modulated radiotherapy for cervical cancer. *Int J Radiat Oncol Biol Phys.* 2007;68(1):166–171.

61. Syed AM, et al. Long-term results of low-dose-rate interstitial-intracavitary brachytherapy in the treatment of carcinoma of the cervix. *Int J Radiat Oncol Biol Phys.* 2002;54(1):67–78.

demos
MEDICAL

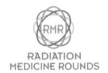

RADIATION
MEDICINE ROUNDS

Intensity-Modulated Radiotherapy in Vulvar Cancer

David A. Clump and Sushil Beriwal*

Department of Radiation Oncology, University of Pittsburgh Cancer Institute, Pittsburgh, PA

■ ABSTRACT

The integration of IMRT into the management of gynecological malignancies including that of vulvar cancer affords an opportunity to deliver the prescription dose in a highly conformal manner, while decreasing dose to nearby surrounding structures. Dosimetric studies that compare IMRT and three-dimensional conformal therapy (3DCRT), clearly demonstrate an ability of this technology to decrease dose to the small bowel, rectum, bladder, bone marrow, and femoral heads while maintaining coverage of the target. The translation of these dosimetric studies into clinical practice offer encouraging preliminary results by maintaining tumor control while potentially reducing treatment-related morbidity. However, the widespread adoption of these techniques is not without the potential for problems as they rely heavily on accurate target delineation and set-up reproducibility. Uniform contouring practices are necessary as multicenter, prospective studies are designed to access the outcomes associated with IMRT. This review focuses on defining the volumes to be treated as well as the organs at risk (OAR) to avoid during the treatment of vulvar cancer.

Keywords: vulvar cancer, IMRT, contouring

■ INTRODUCTION

Cancer of the vulva is the fourth most common gynecological malignancy accounting for about 4000 cases per year in the United States (1). Of those with invasive disease, 30 percent are locally advanced, and radiation therapy (RT) or a combination of chemotherapy and RT is utilized to reduce the volume of disease prior to resection or in select instances as definitive treatment for patients who are not surgical candidates (2). Additionally, adjuvant RT is implemented to improve locoregional control following resection of a bulky primary, in patients who exhibit close or positive margins following resection, as well as in those with inguinal lymph node involvement (3).

With conventional treatment of pelvic malignancies, the primary tumor and draining lymph nodes are irradiated with a uniform radiation dose along with the surrounding normal tissues, including the small bowel, rectum, and bladder. Additional normal tissues including the femoral heads, pelvic bone marrow, and

---

*Corresponding author, Department of Radiation Oncology, University of Pittsburgh Cancer Institute, Pittsburgh, PA 15232
   E-mail address: beriwals@upmc.edu

Radiation Medicine Rounds 2:3 (2011) 383–390.
DOI: 10.5003/2151–4208.2.3.383

uninvolved skin are also affected. In the case of vulvar cancer, conventional 3DCRT consists of an anterior field that treats both the primary tumor and inguinal nodes, while a narrower posterior field encompasses only the primary lesion. To adequately treat the inguinal lymph nodes, supplemental dose is delivered via matched, anterior electron fields, which have the potential of creating significant dose inhomogeneity at the match line. This approach not only presents a dosimetric challenge secondary to its abutting photon–electron field, but also poses the risk of increased skin toxicity as well as toxicity to the aforementioned normal tissues. To reduce dose to the normal structures, as well as to eliminate the challenges associated with abutting fields, modern treatment planning including the introduction of IMRT allows dose to be delivered via multiple noncoplanar fields creating a conformal, relatively homogenous dose distribution which effectively treats the desired target, while minimizing dose to normal surrounding tissues (4).

This optimization in dose distribution is often accomplished via an inverse planning process where the desired dose is prescribed to the volume of interest while limits or constraints are placed upon nearby normal organs and tissues. Following a computer and software facilitated process, beam intensities are adjusted iteratively to achieve an ideal dose distribution that has the potential to reduce toxicity by sparing of normal tissues (4). Despite these advantages, IMRT is not without the potential for a compromise in tumor control as it relies more heavily on accurate target delineation than conventional techniques, including the incorporation of areas at risk for microscopic disease, appreciation of target movement, as well as reproducibility in patient positioning. This report will address these aspects by focusing on the utilization and practical application of IMRT in the management of carcinoma of the vulva.

■ CLINICAL ASSESSMENT

Accurate target delineation is of central importance in delivering effective and safe RT via an IMRT approach. A thorough clinical assessment with examination of the primary and complete gynecological examination to access potential extension of disease, as well as palpation of the inguinal lymph nodes, complements surgical staging in determining the necessity of further work-up and guiding treatment decisions. In the cases with vaginal involvement, a fiducial marker is placed to identify the vaginal

extent of disease. This is helpful not only in target delineation, but also assists in the daily positioning of the patient when image-guidance is utilized.

Physical examination in patients with vulvar carcinoma is neither sensitive nor specific as 25% of patients with clinically enlarged lymph nodes are found to have no evidence of disease on pathologic assessment, while 25% of those with a normal examination are found to have occult metastatic disease (5). Because the most important prognostic factor in patients with vulvar cancer is the presence of lymph node metastases, imaging is essential in guiding therapy. A computed tomography (CT) scan of the abdomen and pelvis is used to access both the primary and nodal status; however, in a retrospective study of 44 patients who underwent a CT scan prior to lymph node dissection, CT had a sensitivity, specificity, negative predictive value (NPV), and positive predictive value (PPV) of 58, 75, 75, and 58%, respectively (6). In contrast, ultrasound combined with final needle aspirate (FNA) cytology had a sensitivity, specificity, NPV, and PPV of 80, 100, 93, and 100% (6).

Advanced imaging techniques, such as positron-emission tomography (PET) and magnetic resonance imaging (MRI), may provide further detail resulting in a modification of the targeted volume and the subsequent dose delivered. Extrapolating from other disease sites within the pelvis, PET-CT can complement the previous examinations and increase the sensitivity of identifying nodal disease that would otherwise be undetected by the combination of physical exam and CT imaging (7). In the case of locally advanced disease, MRI is useful in assessing the relationship between tumor and normal tissues, such as the musculature of the anal sphincter, and vagina (8). Additionally, MRI may be useful in assessing the lymph nodes, as a node greater than 10 mm reflects sensitivity for malignancy of 40% and specificity of 97% (9).

■ IMMOBILIZATION AND TREATMENT PLANNING

For treatment planning purposes, the patient should undergo a CT or PET-CT simulation in the supine position with the lower extremities abducted ("frog-legged") and immobilized in a vacuum-evacuated device to assure reproducibility in set-up. By abducting the lower extremities to the maximal extent allowable by the scanner, dose to the medial thigh and groin folds is minimized. To assist in delineation of the tumor, radiopaque wire is used to identify areas of gross disease or the postoperative tumor bed (Figure 1). Additionally, the CT simulation should be performed with both intravenous and oral contrast, which allows the small bowel, rectum, and bladder to be easily contoured as well as visualization of the vasculature structures. A bolus of 0.5 to 1 cm thickness is usually placed over the vulvar region at the time of treatment planning and during subsequent daily treatments.

■ CONTOURS

Target Volumes

The complement of physical examination and imaging facilitates the identification of the eventual RT target. For vulvar cancer, the gross tumor volume (GTV) is defined as all disease found on examination, palpable lymph nodes, lymph nodes >1.5 cm visualized on CT, and fluorodeoxyglucose (FDG)-positive areas noted on PET-CT. The GTV is expanded by 1 to 2 cm and incorporated into the clinical target volume (CTV), which reflects a combination of the primary site and areas suspected of harboring microscopic disease such as the draining lymph nodes. For vulvar cancer, two CTVs can be created: one to account for the primary disease (CTV1) and the other for the nodal regions

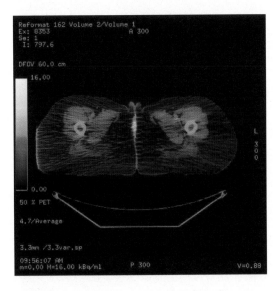

FIGURE 1 The patient is simulated in the supine position on a PET-CT simulator. To assist in target identification, a radiopaque wire is used to identify areas of gross disease.

(CTV2). In general, the CTV1 includes at a minimum the entire vulvar region with a 1-cm margin with careful attention to exclude nearby uninvolved structures such as the muscles comprising the anal sphincter and bone (Figure 2). The CTV is modified by various clinical scenarios, for example, in patients with a posterior vulvar lesion, the CTV1 should also include the perineum from the posterior fourchette to the anal verge. Additionally, in patients with vaginal extension, the CTV1 should include the entire vagina.

The primary pattern of lymph node drainage from the vulva is to the bilateral inguinofemoral lymph nodes; however, the pelvic lymph nodes including the lower common iliac, bilateral external iliac, and internal iliac are also at risk and included in the CTV2. In instances in which there is known disease in the pelvic lymph nodes, the entire common iliac and presacral lymph nodes are also included. To contour the lymph nodes at risk, the pelvic vasculature is used as a surrogate (10). The rationale for this approach is based upon a study by Taylor et al., which identified pelvic lymph nodes following intravenous injection of iron oxide particles with MRI. It was determined that a margin of 7 mm around the vessel accounted for 95% of the common iliac, internal iliac, medial and anterior external iliac, and obturator lymph nodes; however, in the lateral external iliac region and inguinofemoral region, this 7 mm margin on the vessel was not sufficient (11).

The uncertainty in using the vessels as a lymph node surrogate in the inguinofemoral region reflects the variability in the location of the femoral vessels based upon the patient's body habitus and whether a previous dissection of the groin was performed. As a result, the Radiation Therapy Oncology Group (RTOG) recommends contouring the inguinofemoral nodes as a compartment extending caudally about 2 cm from the saphenous-femoral junction to approximately the level of the lesser trochanter (12). In this region, careful attention must be paid to include small vessels and lymph nodes, which subsequently results in an expansion closer to 2 cm on the named vessels. In a preliminary study by Beriwal and colleagues, the relationship between the femoral vessel and positive inguinal lymph nodes was analyzed. Positive inguinofemoral lymph nodes ranged from 0.9 to 3.5 cm from the vessel; therefore, we now contour a region defined laterally by the medial border of the iliopsoas, medially by the lateral border of the adductor longus, posteriorly by the iliopsoas muscle, and pectineus and anteriorly by the edge of the sartorius muscle and rectus femoris (Figure 3) (13).

FIGURE 2 The primary disease, or GTV, is shown in green. To account for microscopic disease, the entire vulva with a margin is included in the clinical target volume-1 (CTV1) (red) with processing to exclude muscle. This volume is then expanded to create the PTV (orange). Note the incorporation of the bolus into the treatment planning software.

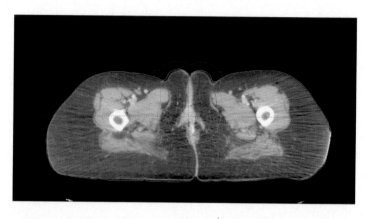

FIGURE 3 A larger expansion on the vessel is needed in the inguinofemoral region to account for potential microscopic involvement. We suggest contouring a region defined laterally by the medial border of the iliopsoas, medially by the lateral border of the adductor longus, posteriorly by the iliopsoas muscle and pectineus, and anteriorly by the edge of the sartorius muscle and rectus femoris.

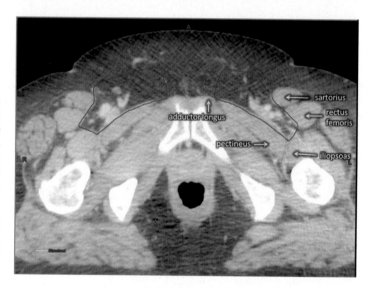

To generate the planning target volume (PTV), the CTVs are expanded to account for variation in patient set-up and motion. Depending upon institutional experience and technology such as linear accelerators equipped with on-board imaging (OBI) and cone-beam CT (CBCT), this expansion is variable. The CTV1 for the primary or tumor bed should be expanded by at least 1 cm to account for the previously mentioned uncertainties; whereas, there is less variation in respect to the lymph nodes and its CTV2 can be expanded by 0.7 to 1.0 cm. Utilizing the Boolean function in the planning software, these volumes are combined to generate the final PTV. This post-expansion volume can then be processed in a manner to spare the skin by 0.5 cm in the inguinal femoral area, whereas the volume is brought to the skin at the primary site.

OAR

In addition to defining the PTV for treatment planning, it is also necessary to identify OAR that serve as avoidance structures in the IMRT optimization process. Of specific interest in vulvar cancer patients undergoing IMRT is constraining dose to the small bowel, rectum, and bladder. There is also potential to spare dose to the femoral heads, pelvic bone marrow, and skin. In general, the entire volume of the rectum including the anal canal is contoured as one structure. Additionally, the entire bladder is contoured in a manner in which there is no overlap between the OAR and CTV. In regard to the small bowel, we advocate contouring the entire peritoneal cavity instead of individual bowel loops and extending contours from the rectosigmoid junction to 1 to 2 cm above the PTV. With respect to the femoral heads, the contours are continued caudally to the level of the lesser trochanter. In instances in which chemotherapy is given concurrent with radiotherapy, the pelvic bone marrow should be included as a constraint when the patient is at increased risk for hematologic sequelae. As 50% of the total bone marrow reserve is located within the pelvis, the pelvic bones including the lower lumbar spine, iliac, sacrum, and femoral heads can serve as a surrogate and be contoured as an avoidance structure (14,15).

IMRT Planning and Dose Selection

Following identification of the target volume and OARs as described, input parameters for IMRT planning of the PTV are typically as follows: ≤35% of the small bowel to receive ≥35.0 Gy (maximum dose: 50.0 Gy); ≤40% of the bladder to receive ≥40 Gy (maximum dose: 50.0 Gy); ≤40% of the rectum to receive ≥40.0 Gy (maximum dose: 50.0 Gy); ≤35% of the femoral heads to receive ≥35.0 Gy (maximum dose: 50.0 Gy); ≤80% of the pelvic bone marrow to receive ≥20.0 Gy (maximum dose: 50.0 Gy) (16). The IMRT plans are optimized to minimize the volume of PTV receiving <95% or >110% of the prescribed dose (Figure 4). The bolus should be integrated into the IMRT treatment plan and at the time of the first treatment, a thermoluminescent dosimeter (TLD) should be placed under the bolus to confirm the prescribed dose.

In the adjuvant setting, the prescribed dose is 45 to 50.4 Gy with additional boost to areas of positive margin and/or extracapsular extension to a total dose of 55 to 60 Gy. Similarly, the dose for preoperative chemoradiation treatment of vulvar cancer is usually 45 to 50.4 Gy delivered via conventional fractionation or a hybrid hyperfractionated regimen

(17–19). The patient may get an additional boost to the primary site and involved lymph nodes if RT is used as definitive treatment. Depending on response, the total dose in this instance is 60 to 70 Gy.

As will be discussed in greater detail below, IMRT reduces dose to the normal surrounding tissues; therefore, creating the possibility for dose escalation. In patients treated definitively with a sequential IMRT boost, it is imperative to rescan the patient to account for tumor response and subsequent adjustment of the targeted volume. In regard to the nodal GTV, this volume is expanded 0.5 to 1.0 cm to create the final nodal boost volume, while the primary GTV is expanded by 1 to 2 cm. The boost to the primary site can be delivered via an IMRT plan or a direct electron field depending on the response and location of remaining disease.

An alternative approach for treating gross nodal disease is the delivery of a simultaneous integrated boost (SIB) during the initial 45.0 Gy delivered to the pelvis. In this approach, a portion of the target, such as a positive inguinal lymph node, is treated at a higher dose per fraction than that of areas harboring microscopic disease. At the University of Pittsburgh, we use a total of 55 Gy delivered at 2.2 Gy per fraction to the positive lymph node plus a 1.0-cm margin, while the areas at risk for microscopic disease receive 45 Gy delivered at 1.8 Gy per fraction. The advantage of this technique is that dose can be escalated without increasing the overall treatment time.

Image-Guided Radiotherapy

Assuring accurate dose delivery is essential for the success of IMRT in treating vulvar cancer. In patients with disease extension to the vagina,

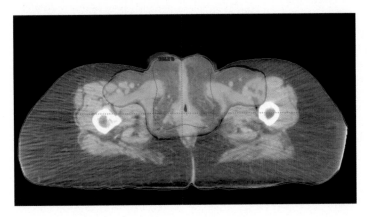

FIGURE 4 IMRT facilitates the delivery of a relatively homogenous dose to the target while optimizing the beam arrangement to reduce dose to normal surrounding structures. It is feasible to bring the prescribed dose to the surface at the primary site with use of a bolus or in the case of the inguinal region, spare the skin to reduce toxicity.

the bladder-filling position can cause significant motion of the vaginal apex. One way to account for this variation is to perform a CT scan with a full and empty bladder, thus creating an internal target volume (ITV) for the vaginal region. It is recommended that the patient be treated with a full bladder; however, its reproducibility is difficult to ensure. OBI with kilovoltage (kV) imaging can also be used daily to reduce interfractional motion as adjustments can be based on the bony anatomy or on fiducial markers placed at the vaginal extent of disease (if present). Additionally, CBCT can be used to assure that the patient is in the correct treatment position.

■ DOSIMETRIC STUDIES

Using similar input factors for PTV planning, the dosimetric advantages of IMRT over that of 3DCRT have been described for the management of gynecological malignancies (14,16,20–22). By comparing treatment plans and dose volume histograms (DVH) generated for patients receiving adjuvant RT for cervical and endometrial cancer, the volume of small bowel, rectum, and bladder receiving >30 Gy (V_{30}) are reduced by 52, 66, and 36%, respectively, when IMRT compared with 3DCRT (20). Likewise, in patients with vulvar cancer where the target includes not only the vulva and pelvic nodes, but also the inguinal lymph node region, IMRT has been shown to reduce the V_{30} of small bowel, rectum, and bladder by 27, 41, and 26%, respectively, compared with conventional 3DCRT (16).

Additional studies have demonstrated the feasibility of dose reduction to the pelvic bone marrow and femoral heads, which in turn creates the opportunity to reduce toxicity by modulating the amount of dose delivered to these structures (14,22). Reduction of hematologic toxicity, by using a dosimetric model wherein bone-marrow sparing (BMS)-IMRT and a four-field box technique, IMRT planning was proven more effective at reducing the volume of pelvic bone marrow receiving dose >16.4 Gy, while also maintaining a lower dose than conventional techniques to the small bowel (14). These data support the concept of using IMRT to significantly reduce toxicity when compared with conventional techniques in the treatment of carcinoma of the vulva.

■ CLINICAL IMPLEMENTATION

Adjuvant RT

Following surgical intervention for vulva cancer, the pathological findings of grossly positive nodes, ≥2 lymph nodes positive, and ≥20% of ipsilateral lymph nodes being positive dictate the necessity of adjuvant RT and the potential for the implementation of IMRT (23,24). While clinical data supporting the use of IMRT in the adjuvant setting of vulvar cancer is limited, the lymph node volumes targeted by RT place the patient at risk for significant toxicity to the small bowel, rectum, and bladder. This risk is similar to other gynecologic and pelvic malignancies in which data exist.

Utilizing IMRT, Mundt and coworkers reported the side-effect profile of 40 patients treated for gynecological malignancies compared with a matched cohort receiving conventional treatment. In this study, patients treated with IMRT experienced less grade 2 or higher acute gastrointestinal toxicity (60 vs. 91%, $p < .002$) when compared with conventional 3DCRT (25). This likely reflected the decrease in the volume of bowel treated in comparison with conventional therapy as IMRT reduced the volume of bowel treated from 600 to 300 cc (26). In a dosimetric and early outcomes analysis, Beriwal and colleagues reported the feasibility and results of implementing IMRT in the adjuvant setting of eight patients with vulvar cancer. In this subset, there were no reports of grade 3 gastrointestinal toxicity and all patients completed treatment without interruption (16).

Despite initial controversy regarding the effectiveness of RT in lieu of surgery in treating the inguinal nodal region, its efficacy has since been validated provided that dose is prescribed to an adequate depth and volume (27). Treatment of the inguinal lymph nodes with a conventional 3DCRT set-up and a matched anterior electron field involves multiple challenges, including dose inhomogeneity of dose at the match line which reflects the abutting photon–electron fields. Additionally, the patient is positioned isocentrically during the delivery of the pelvic field, while the matched, direct electron field is delivered via a source-skin distance (SSD) set-up, which requires the therapist to enter room and make corresponding adjustments resulting in increased potential for set-up uncertainty. With its isocentric set-up and its mode of delivery, IMRT has the potential to decrease the risk of set-up uncertainties and also produce a relatively homogenous dose distribution.

An additional concern with the direct electron field is that adequate dose delivery to the inguinal region requires the selection of high-energy electrons to treat inguinal nodal depths that are often >5 cm. Despite its effectiveness, there is the potential for acute grade 3 skin toxicity to the medial thigh and groin folds. With IMRT and the use of photons the potential skin toxicity is less. In a similarly treated cancer (anal cancer), grade 3 and 4 dermatologic toxicity was approximately 50% with conventional techniques; yet, with the implementation of IMRT this toxicity compared favorably to historical controls occurring at a rate of 20 to 25% (28,29). A similar reduction in toxicity would be expected when IMRT is used for the treatment of vulvar cancer.

Locally Advanced Disease

In addition to adjuvant treatment, RT is used in instances in which radical surgical excision of the vulva is not sufficient to remove the cancer with adequate margins or instances in which a pelvic exenteration is required. Since there is significant physical and psychological morbidity resulting from these procedures, preoperative chemoradiation is an accepted alternative to treat these patients. There have been multiple phase II and single institution studies showing the efficacy of this approach including one of which that utilized IMRT (17–19).

Employing a preoperative regimen similar to the Gynecologic Oncology Group (GOG) 101 study, a hybrid hyperfractionation regimen with IMRT concurrent with cisplatin and 5-fluorouracil (5-FU) has been described (19). The radiation schema consisted of 1.6 Gy twice a day for 10 fractions, followed by 1.8 to 2 Gy once a day for 7 to 8 fractions, followed by a planned break of 10 days and then resumption of radiation with 1.6 Gy twice a day for 10 more fractions (19). With a median follow-up of 22 months, 14 of 18 patients underwent surgical resection, of which 9 had a complete pathological response (pCR), and a resulting specific and overall survival of 75 and 70%, respectively. Overall the treatment was well tolerated with no significant grade 3 morbidity. All patients exhibited acute desquamative skin reactions in the vulva and perineum. However, none experienced moist desquamation in the groin (19).

■ CONCLUSIONS

The integration of IMRT into the management of gynecological malignancies including that of vulvar cancer provides an opportunity to deliver the prescription dose in a conformal, relatively homogenous manner while eliminating the dosimetric and technical challenges associated with conventional treatment. By shaping the dose to the target in 3D, there is also the potential for a decrease in the morbidity associated with treatment. This is supported by preclinical models that compare IMRT and 3DCRT wherein there is clear demonstration of the ability of this technology to decrease dose to critical normal structures including the small bowel, rectum, bladder, pelvic bone marrow, and femoral heads, while maintaining coverage of the target. While the clinical outcome data regarding the use of IMRT in the management of vulvar cancer remains limited, there are encouraging preliminary studies from both the gynecological literature as well as that of other pelvic malignancies including anal cancer that support its use.

Despite its potential, the widespread adoption of these techniques is not without potential for complications as this technology relies heavily on accurate target delineation and set-up reproducibility. Uniform contouring practices are necessary as multicenter, prospective studies are designed to access the outcomes associated with IMRT. This review focused primarily on the manner of defining the volumes to be treated as well as the OAR that are capable of being avoided. Future studies will likely focus on delivering higher than conventional doses to areas of gross disease via a SIB or dose-painting approach while continuing to reduce inter- and intrafractional uncertainties.

■ REFERENCES

1. Jemal A, Siegel R, Xu J, et al. Cancer statistics, 2010. *CA Cancer J Clin.* 2010;60:277–300.

2. Stroup AM, Harlan LC, Trimble EL. Demographic, clinical, and treatment trends among women diagnosed with vulvar cancer in the United States. *Gynecol Oncol.* 2008;108:577–583.

3. Perez CA, Grigsby PW, Galakatos A, et al. Radiation therapy in management of carcinoma of the vulva with emphasis on conservation therapy. *Cancer.* 1993;71:3707–3716.

4. Intensity modulated radiation therapy collaborative working group. Current status and issues of interest. *Int J Radiat Oncol Biol Phys.* 2001;51:880–914.

5. Montana GS, Kang SK. Carcinoma of the vulva. In: Perez CA, Brady LW, Halperin EW, et al., eds. *Principles and Practice of Radiation Oncology.* 4th ed. Philadelphia: Lippincott Williams & Wilkins; 2004;2003–2022.

6. Land R, Herod J, Moskovic E, et al. Routine computerized tomography scanning, groin ultrasound with or without fine needle aspiration cytology in the surgical management of primary squamous cell carcinoma of the vulva. *Int J Gynecol Cancer.* 2006;16:312–317.

7. Cotter SE, Grigsby PW, Siegel BA, et al. FDG-PET/CT in the evaluation of anal carcinoma. *Int J Radiat Oncol Biol Phys.* 2006;65:720–725.

8. Griffin N, Grant LA, Sala E. Magnetic resonance imaging of vaginal and vulval pathology. *Eur Radiol.* 2008;18:1269–1280.

9. Sohaib SA, Moskovic EC. Imaging in vulval cancer. *Best Pract Res Clin Obstet Gynaecol.* 2003;17:543–556.

10. Small W, Jr., Mell LK, Anderson P, et al. Consensus guidelines for delineation of clinical target volume for intensity-modulated pelvic radiotherapy in postoperative treatment of endometrial and cervical cancer. *Int J Radiat Oncol Biol Phys.* 2008;71:428–434.

11. Taylor A, Rockall AG, Reznek RH, et al. Mapping pelvic lymph nodes: guidelines for delineation in intensity-modulated radiotherapy. *Int J Radiat Oncol Biol Phys.* 2005;63:1604–1612.

12. Myerson RJ, Garofalo MC, El Naga I, et al. Elective clinical target volumes for conformal therapy in anorectal cancer: A radiation therapy oncology group consensus panel contouring atlas. *Int J Radiat Oncol Biol Phys.* 2009;74:824–830.

13. Beriwal S, Kim CH, Olson AC. *Guidelines for defining clinical target volumes in contouring inguinal and femoral lymph nodes in intensity modulated radiation therapy.* Presented at the 53rd Annual Meeting of the American Society of Radiation Oncology (ASTRO) Miami, FL, 2011.

14. Mell LK, Tiryaki H, Ahn KH, et al. Dosimetric comparison of bone marrow-sparing intensity-modulated radiotherapy versus conventional techniques for treatment of cervical cancer. *Int J Radiat Oncol Biol Phys.* 2008;71:1504–1510.

15. Ellis RE. The distribution of active bone marrow in the adult. *Phys Med Biol.* 1961;5:255–258.

16. Beriwal S, Heron DE, Kim H, et al. Intensity-modulated radiotherapy for the treatment of vulvar carcinoma: A comparative dosimetric study with early clinical outcome. *Int J Radiat Oncol Biol Phys.* 2006;64:1395–1400.

17. Montana GS, Thomas GM, Moore DH, et al. Preoperative chemo-radiation for carcinoma of the vulva with N2/N3 nodes: A gynecologic oncology group study. *Int J Radiat Oncol Biol Phys.* 2000;48:1007–1013.

18. Moore DH, Thomas GM, Montana GS, et al. Preoperative chemoradiation for advanced vulvar cancer: A phase II study of the Gynecologic Oncology Group. *Int J Radiat Oncol Biol Phys.* 1998;42:79–85.

19. Beriwal S, Coon D, Heron DE, et al. Preoperative intensity-modulated radiotherapy and chemotherapy for locally advanced vulvar carcinoma. *Gynecol Oncol.* 2008;109:291–295.

20. Heron DE, Gerszten K, Selvaraj RN, et al. Conventional 3D conformal versus intensity-modulated radiotherapy for the adjuvant treatment of gynecologic malignancies: A comparative dosimetric study of dose-volume histograms small star, filled. *Gynecol Oncol.* 2003;91:39–45.

21. Roeske JC, Lujan A, Rotmensch J, et al. Intensity-modulated whole pelvic radiation therapy in patients with gynecologic malignancies. *Int J Radiat Oncol Biol Phys.* 2000;48:1613–1621.

22. Gilroy JS, Amdur RJ, Louis DA, et al. Irradiating the groin nodes without breaking a leg: A comparison of techniques for groin node irradiation. *Med Dosim.* 2004;29:258–264.

23. Homesley HD, Bundy BN, Sedlis A, et al. Radiation therapy versus pelvic node resection for carcinoma of the vulva with positive groin nodes. *Obstet Gynecol.* 1986;68:733–740.

24. Kunos C, Simpkins F, Gibbons H, et al. Radiation therapy compared with pelvic node resection for node-positive vulvar cancer: A randomized controlled trial. *Obstet Gynecol.* 2009;114:537–546.

25. Mundt AJ, Lujan AE, Rotmensch J, et al. Intensity-modulated whole pelvic radiotherapy in women with gynecologic malignancies. *Int J Radiat Oncol Biol Phys.* 2002;52:1330–1337.

26. Mundt AJ, Roeske JC, Lujan AE. Intensity-modulated radiation therapy in gynecologic malignancies. *Med Dosim.* 2002;27:131–136.

27. Stehman FB, Bundy BN, Thomas G, et al. Groin dissection versus groin radiation in carcinoma of the vulva: a Gynecologic Oncology Group study. *Int J Radiat Oncol Biol Phys.* 1992;24:389–396.

28. Ajani JA, Winter KA, Gunderson LL, et al. Fluorouracil, mitomycin, and radiotherapy vs fluorouracil, cisplatin, and radiotherapy for carcinoma of the anal canal: a randomized controlled trial. *JAMA.* 2008;299:1914–1921.

29. Kachnic LA, Tsai HK, Coen JJ, et al. Dose-painted intensity-modulated radiation therapy for anal cancer: a multi-institutional report of acute toxicity and response to therapy. *Int J Radiat Oncol Biol Phys.* 2011 (in press).

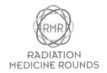

RADIATION
MEDICINE ROUNDS

Chemotherapy in Advanced/Recurrent Endometrial Cancer

Vicky Makker*

Gynecologic Medical Oncology Service, Memorial Sloan-Kettering Cancer Center, New York, NY

■ ABSTRACT

Most endometrial cancer patients are diagnosed with early stage disease and have favorable outcomes. In contrast, the subset of women presenting with advanced/recurrent disease have a poor prognosis and represent a therapeutic challenge. In this review, clinical trials of chemotherapy in endometrial cancer patients with advanced and/or recurrent disease are reviewed. The rationale for hormonal therapy and its efficacy in this patient population are also presented. Finally, the development of novel biologic and targeted agents in advanced/recurrent disease patients is reviewed along with the results of early clinical trials focused on these agents.

Keywords: advanced, endometrial, chemotherapy, targeted therapy

■ INTRODUCTION

Endometrial cancer is the most common gynecologic malignancy in the United States, with an annual incidence of 40,000 cases (1). The majority of patients are diagnosed with early stage cancer, which is typically treated surgically with overall excellent outcomes. However, patients with recurrent disease or metastatic disease have incurable disease with limited treatment options and poor prognosis. Such patients account for the approximately 8,000 annual deaths from this cancer (1).

Investigations focusing on new approaches to improve outcomes in patients with advanced/recurrent disease are warranted. There have been multiple randomized studies performed by the Gynecologic Oncology Group (GOG) addressing the issue of optimal therapy for this group of patients. Once this initial therapy has been delivered, either in the adjuvant or advanced disease setting, there are limited treatment options, with no standard options available.

■ ADJUVANT THERAPY: ADVANCED DISEASE

The optimal adjuvant treatment strategy for patients presenting with advanced stage endometrial cancer is still not well-defined. In the past, surgical resection has been followed by pelvic or whole-abdominal

*Corresponding author, Gynecologic Medical Oncology Service, Memorial Sloan-Kettering Cancer, 1275 York Avenue, New York, NY 10065
    E-mail address: makkerv@mskcc.org

Radiation Medicine Rounds 2:3 (2011) 391–400.
DOI: 10.5003/2151–4208.2.3.391

radiotherapy (WART). However, systemic failures outside the treatment field have limited the impact of radiotherapy (RT) on long-term patient survival. In recent years, chemotherapy has demonstrated significant activity in women with advanced endometrial cancer and has become the standard treatment. Its benefits rely on the sterilization of systemic foci of metastatic disease. However, if chemotherapy is delivered alone, the crude proportion of patients with pelvic recurrences (18%), abdominal recurrences (14%), and extra-abdominal or liver metastases (18%) is high, which can ultimately lead to systemic recurrence and death (2). Investigators have thus hypothesized that a combined approach (chemotherapy plus RT) may provide better disease control, by preventing both local/pelvic recurrences, as well as failure in distant sites, as opposed to chemotherapy alone.

GOG 122 was a randomized phase III trial of WART versus doxorubicin-cisplatin chemotherapy in women with advanced endometrial carcinoma (2). In this study, 422 patients with stage III/IV disease of any histology were entered; of the 396 assessable patients, 202 received WART, and 194 received doxorubicin-cisplatin. The radiation dose was 30 Gy in 20 fractions, with a 15-Gy pelvic boost. Chemotherapy consisted of doxorubicin (60 mg/m^2) and cisplatin (50 mg/m^2) every 3 weeks for seven cycles, followed by one cycle of cisplatin. All patients underwent total abdominal hysterectomy, bilateral salpingo-oophorectomy, and staging. Pelvic and paraaortic lymph node dissection was optional, and no single site of residual disease >2 cm was allowed. Treatment had to begin within 8 weeks of surgery. The median patient age was 63 years; 50% of patients had endometrioid tumors and 73% had stage III disease. At a median follow-up of 74 months, the hazard ratio (HR) for progression (adjusted for stage) was 0.71, favoring adjuvant chemotherapy (95% confidence interval [CI], 0.55–0.91; $p < .01$). The stage-adjusted death HR was 0.68 (95% CI, 0.52–0.89; $p < .01$), also favoring doxorubicin-cisplatin (2).

GOG 184 randomized advanced endometrial carcinoma patients following surgery and volume-directed RT to six cycles of cisplatin (50 mg/m^2) and doxorubicin (45 mg/m^2) with or without paclitaxel (160 mg/m^2) (3). In this study, all patients underwent surgical debulking (optional lymph node sampling). Those with stage III/IV (66 stage IV patients randomized; June 2003 closed to stage IV patients) disease with <2 cm disease were eligible, and received volume-directed RT to the pelvis/paraaortic lymph

nodes. Radiation treatment had to begin within 8 weeks following surgery, and chemotherapy had to begin within 8 weeks following RT.

Of 659 women enrolled, 552 eligible patients were randomized to chemotherapy following RT. The percentage of patients alive and recurrence-free at 36 months was 62% for cisplatin-doxorubicin versus 64% for cisplatin-doxorubicin-paclitaxel. Tumor stage, residual disease, histology/grade, positive paraaortic node and cytology, pelvic metastases and age were significantly associated with recurrence-free survival. This study revealed that the addition of paclitaxel to cisplatin and doxorubicin following surgery and volume-directed RT was not associated with a significant improvement in recurrence-free survival, but was associated with increased toxicity (3).

The Radiation Therapy Oncology Group (RTOG) trial 9708 evaluated adjuvant postoperative RT combined with cisplatin/paclitaxel chemotherapy following surgery in patients with high-risk endometrial cancer (grade 2 or 3 endometrial adenocarcinoma with >50% myometrial invasion, stromal invasion of the cervix, or pelvic-confined extrauterine disease) (4). This study was designed to administer 45 Gy in 25 fractions to the pelvis, along with cisplatin (50 mg/m^2) on days 1 and 28. Vaginal brachytherapy with a low-dose-rate applicator (20 Gy to the surface) or high-dose-rate applicator (6 Gy × 3 to the surface) was performed after external beam RT. Four courses of cisplatin (50 mg/m^2) and paclitaxel (175 mg/m^2) were administered at 4-week intervals after the completion of RT. Overall, 42 patients were evaluated. Follow-up ranged from 6.9 to 48.8 months (median, 28.7 months). At 24 months, the pelvic and distant recurrence rates were 2% and 17%, respectively. Corresponding disease-free and overall survivals were 83% and 90%, respectively (4).

Building on the experience of the GOG and RTOG, GOG 258 is a currently open randomized phase III trial of cisplatin and volume-directed RT followed by carboplatin and paclitaxel versus carboplatin and paclitaxel alone for optimally debulked, advanced endometrial carcinoma. In this study, patients with stage III/IV disease are randomized to cisplatin (50 mg/m^2 on days 1 and 29) plus volume-directed RT followed by carboplatin (AUC 5) plus paclitaxel (175 mg/m^2 every 21 days for 4 cycles) versus carboplatin (AUC 6) plus paclitaxel (175 mg/m^2 every 21 days for 6 cycles). The aim of the trial is to determine if treatment with cisplatin and volume-directed RT followed by carboplatin and paclitaxel for 4 cycles (experimental arm) reduces the rate of recurrence or death (i.e., increases recurrence-free survival) when compared with chemotherapy consisting of carboplatin and paclitaxel for six cycles (control arm) in patients with Stages III–IVA endometrial carcinoma (<2 cm residual disease).

It is now clear that systemic chemotherapy should be part of the treatment for advanced stage endometrial cancer patients. It is also predicted that RT will decrease the rate of local failure. However, it is not known whether the addition of volume-directed RT to chemotherapy alters recurrence-free and overall survivals in a significant manner. GOG 258 is the logical follow-up to the previous research questions addressed by earlier GOG protocols (122, 184, and 209). This trial will answer critical questions regarding (a) the impact of chemoradiation in this setting, (b) the tolerability of this approach compared with the standard of care, and (c) the short- and long-term impact of combined treatment on the quality of life. A positive trial would lead to a new standard treatment that could easily be adopted in the community.

■ HORMONAL THERAPY IN ADVANCED/RECURRENT ENDOMETRIAL CANCER: NO PRIOR CHEMOTHERAPY

Steroid hormones play an important role in the control of normal and malignant endometrium. Endometrial carcinoma has been recognized for many years as a hormonally sensitive neoplasm. Medroxyprogesterone acetate (MPA) is a synthetic progestin with antiestrogenic properties, which disrupt the estrogen receptor cycle. MPA is an anti-neoplastic progestin that interferes with the normal estrogen cycle and results in lower leutenizing hormone levels. This may have a direct effect on the endometrium and may act through an antileutenizing effect medicated via the pituitary gland. As seen in laboratory studies, MPA also results in down-regulation of progestin-one receptors, possibly explaining the short response duration (5,6). Estrogen receptor alpha appears to play an important role in regulating progesterone receptors (7).

Although tamoxifen is both an estrogen antagonist and agonist in the body, it is estrogenic in the endometrium, where it binds to estrogen receptors, translocates with the receptor complex to the nucleus, and increases the expression of progesterone receptors by activating transcription of this estrogen responsive gene. By this method, tamoxifen may increase progesterone responsiveness by allowing progestins to further destroy cancer cells (8).

Down-regulation of progesterone receptors is seen in animal studies, possibly explaining the short response duration. Intermittent progestin administration has been suggested, possibly with the addition of tamoxifen to increase the duration and magnitude of response in patients with endometrial cancer (9).

Tamoxifen binds with cytosolic estrogen receptors and translocates with the reception to the nucleus, without exhibiting a typical estrogen response. This receptor-complex increases cytosolic progesterone receptors and decreases cytosolic estrogen receptors, suggesting activity in the treatment of endometrial cancer (8,9).

Alternating treatment strategy of alternating MPA with tamoxifen is felt to lead to a destroy malignant cells-recruit receptors-destroy malignant cells paradigm, and thereby treating the patient. This strategy may prolong MPA responsiveness in endometrial cancer cells by using tamoxifen to counterbalance the MPA-induced down-regulation of progesterone receptor levels, allowing the possibility of endometrial cancer cells to respond to MPA by undergoing differentiation and/or apoptosis.

Response rates to hormonal therapies in advanced uterine cancer are shown in Table 1 (10–15). Megestrol acetate (MA) was approved by the Food and Drug Administration in 1971 for the palliative treatment of advanced, recurrent, inoperable, and metastatic carcinoma of the breast and endometrium. When given to chemotherapy-naive patients, hormonal therapy can result in response rates of up to 33%, but responses are of short duration (median progression-free survival of 2.5 to 3.2 months). Also, these agents are most effective in grade 1 and 2 endometrioid cancers (Table 2) (10–15).

■ HEMOTHERAPY IN ADVANCED/ RECURRENT ENDOMETRIAL CANCER

Patients with recurrent or metastatic endometrial carcinoma often receive hormonal therapy. Although hormonal therapy offers effective palliation in the minority of women with well-differentiated tumors

TABLE 1 Hormonal treatment in advanced endometrial cancer

Study	n	Treatment	RR (%)	PFS (mos)	OS (mos)
GOG 153 (10)	56	MA 80 mg bid × 3 weeks alternating with T 20 mg bid × 3 weeks	27	2.7	14
GOG 121 (11)	58	MA 800 mg daily	24	2.5	7.6
GOG 81 (12)	154	MPA 1,000 mg daily versus	14	2.5	7
	145	MPA 200 mg daily	25	3.2	11.1
GOG 119 (13)	58	T 20 mg bid plus MPA 100 mg bid every other week	33	3	13
GOG 81F (14)	68	T 20 mg bid	10	1.9	8.8
GOG 168 (15)	23	Anastrozole 1 mg daily	9	1	6

OS, overall survival; PFS, progression-free survival; GOG, Gynecologic Oncology Group; MA, megesterol acetate; MPA, medroxyprogesterone acetate; T, tamoxifen; RR, response rate.

TABLE 2 Response rates to hormonal treatment in advanced stage endometrial cancer patients

Study	n	Treatment	Response Rates (%)		
			Grade 1	Grade 2	Grade 3
GOG 153 (10)	56	MA 80 mg bid × 3 weeks alternating with T 20 mg bid × 3 weeks	38 (n = 16)	24 (n = 17)	22 (n = 23)
GOG 121 (11)	58	MA 800 mg daily	37	37	8
GOG 81 (12)	154	MPA 1,000 mg daily	37	23	9
	145	MPA 200 mg daily			
GOG 119 (13)	58	T 20 mg bid plus MPA 100 mg bid every other week	–	–	–
GOG 81F (14)	68	T 20 mg bid	23	14	3
GOG 168 (15)	23	Anastrozole 1 mg daily	–	22 (n = 9)	0 (n = 14)

OS, overall survival; PFS, progression-free survival; RR, response rate; T, tamoxifen.

or tumors expressing high levels of the progesterone receptor, for the majority of patients, hormonal therapy offers only modest benefits, albeit with minimal toxicities.

Single-Agent Studies: No Prior Chemotherapy

For patients whose cancer is refractory to hormonal therapy, treatment with cytotoxic agents has been attempted. As seen in Table 3, only a handful of agents have demonstrated reproducible response rates ≥20%. These agents include doxorubicin (16), cisplatin (17), carboplatin (18,19), paclitaxel (20), ifosfamide (21), topotecan (22), and liposomal doxorubicin (Doxil) (23).

TABLE 3 Endometrial cancer: Single agents with no prior chemotherapy

Agent	RR (%)	References
Doxorubicin	37	16
Cisplatin	20	17
Carboplatin	28	18
	30	19
Paclitaxel	36	20
Ifosfamide	24	21
Topotecan	20	22
Doxil	11.5	23

RR, response rate.

Phase II Studies

The GOG has conducted a series of phase II studies in patients with recurrent/advanced endometrial cancer. In these trials, all histologic subtypes were eligible, but patients must have measurable disease and have had one prior chemotherapy regimen for the treatment of their malignancy. The results of these studies are summarized in Table 4 (24–29). It is evident that even with one prior chemotherapy regimen, response rates to subsequent regimens declines significantly.

Phase III Studies

In an effort to determine the optimal chemotherapy combination for patients with advanced/recurrent endometrial cancer, GOG 107 randomized 281 women to doxorubicin alone (60 mg/m^2) versus doxorubicin (60 mg/m^2) plus cisplatin (50 mg/m^2) (30). A statistically significant advantage to combination therapy was noted with regard to response rate (25% vs. 42%; p = .004) and progression-free survival (3.8 vs. 5.7 months; HR 0.74; 95% CI 0.58, 0.94; p = .14), although no difference in overall survival was observed (9 vs. 9.2 months).

Coincident with the planning of the subsequent GOG trial, phase II data demonstrated that paclitaxel had significant single-agent activity with a response rate of 36% in advanced or recurrent endometrial cancer. Thus, 317 patients were randomized to paclitaxel and doxorubicin or the standard arm of doxorubicin-cisplatin in GOG 163 (30). However, this trial failed to demonstrate a significant difference in response rates, progression-free or overall survivals between the two arms, and doxorubicin-cisplatin remained the standard of care.

Since both platinum and paclitaxel had demonstrated high single-agent activity, there was strong interest in including paclitaxel and cisplatin in a front-line regimen for advanced and recurrent endometrial cancer. Subsequently, GOG 177 randomized 263 women to doxorubicin-cisplatin versus doxorubicin-cisplatin-paclitaxel. Doxorubicin (45 mg/m^2) and cisplatin (50 mg/m^2) were administered on day 1, followed by paclitaxel (160 mg/m^2 over 3 h) on day 2 (with growth factor support) (31). Doxorubicin-cisplatin-paclitaxel was found to be superior in terms of overall response rate (57% vs. 34%; p < .01), median progression-free survival (8.3 vs. 5.3 months; p < .01) and median overall survival (15.3 vs. 12.3 months; p = .037) (32). This improved efficacy came at the cost of increased toxicity. More recently, in GOG 209 doxorubicin-cisplatin-paclitaxel was compared with paclitaxel and carboplatin in an attempt to address this issue. GOG 209 completed accrual April 20, 2009 and is under follow-up.

Given these studies, first-line treatment for metastatic or recurrent disease remains a combination regimen of a platinum agent with either a taxane, anthracycline or both. However, once this initial therapy has been delivered, either in the adjuvant or advanced disease setting, there are limited treatment options, with no established standard options available.

■ DEVELOPMENTAL THERAPEUTICS IN ADVANCED/RECURRENT ENDOMETRIAL CANCER

Most patients with recurrent disease will not be cured by salvage therapy and a series of biologic and targeted agents in recurrent endometrial cancer are

TABLE 4   Phase II studies

Study	Agent	n	RR (%)
GOG 129C (24)	Paclitaxel	44	27.3[a]
GOG 129H (25)	Liposomal doxorubicin	42	9.5
GOG 129J (26)	Topotecan	22	9
GOG 129K (27)	Oxaliplatin	52	13.5
GOG 129N (28)	Docetaxel (weekly)	26	7.7[b]
GOG 129P (29)	Ixabepilone	50	12[c]

RR, response rate.
[a]No prior taxane allowed; [b]77% (20/26) prior paclitaxel; [c]94% (47/50) prior paclitaxel.

being evaluated by the GOG in Phase II studies. Patients entering these trials must have measurable disease and have had either one prior chemotherapy treatment or 1 or 2 prior chemotherapy treatments. Thus far, trastuzumab (GOG 181B), thalidomide (GOG 229B), gefitinib (GOG 229C), GW-572016 (lapatinib, GOG 229D), the anti-VEGF ligand compound bevacizumab (GOG 229E), aflibercept (GOG 229F), bevacizumab/temsirolimus (GOG 229G), AZD6244 (GOG 229H), Brivanib (GOG 229I) cediranib (GOG 229J), and AMG386 (GOG 229L) have been studied or are still accruing patients.

Angiogenesis is one of the cardinal processes leading to invasion and metastasis of solid tumors. The angiogenic-signaling pathway may be triggered by the release of angiogenic promoters, such as vascular endothelial growth factor (VEGF), from tumor cells into the local microenvironment. There is evidence that angiogenesis plays a role in endometrial cancer disease progression and prognosis.

A phase II GOG study of thalidomide in refractory endometrial cancer demonstrated an association between elevated plasma VEGF levels and poor prognosis (33). VEGF receptor (VEGFR) was found to be present in up to two-thirds of endometrial adenocarcinoma specimens (34), and VEGF expression was higher in endometrial adenocarcinoma than in normally cycling endometrium (35). VEGFR-2(flk-1) and VEGFR-3 were found to be poor prognostic factors in endometrial cancer (36,37). VEGF-A/VEGF-1 expression has also been shown to be associated with decreased 5- and 10-year disease-free survivals in postmenopausal patients with endometrial carcinoma (38). Further study of the VEGF, VEGF-R(KDR) pathway in stage I endometrial carcinoma demonstrated a worse prognosis for tumors bearing activated KDR (pKDR) (39). This study identified pKDR in endometrial cancer, endothelial and stromal cells. pKDR levels correlated with KDR/VEGF complex levels. Of note, KDR activation was also associated with an elevation with HIF-1alpha, an up-regulator of VEGF. These relationships point to a VEGF autocrine loop, which can serve as a therapeutic target.

Single-agent bevacizumab has been studied by the GOG in study 229E (40). Eligible women had persistent or recurrent disease after receiving one or two prior cytotoxic regimens, measurable disease, and GOG performance status of <2. Treatment consisted of bevacizumab (15 mg/kg every 3 weeks) until disease progression or prohibitive toxicity. Primary endpoints were progression-free survival at 6 months,

objective response rate, and toxicity. This trial was carried out in a flexible 2-stage group sequential design intended to detect either cytostatic or cytotoxic activity. Median patient age was 62 (range, 44–84) years, and prior treatment consisted of 1 or 2 regimens in 33 and 20 patients, respectively. Twenty-eight women (52.8%) had prior RT. The response rate was 13%, with a 6-month progression-free survival of 40%.

GOG 229G, a phase II evaluation of combination bevacizumab and temsirolimus in the treatment of recurrent of persistent endometrial cancer, revealed that 11 patients (22.9%) had a partial or complete response (90% CI: 13.4%, 35.1%). Twenty-two patients (45.8%) had a progression-free survival of ≥6 months (90% CI: 33.4%, 58.6%). The median progression-free survival was 5.5 months (first and third quartiles were 3.6 and 11.3 months, respectively). Median overall survival was 13.4 months (first quartile was 7.8 months). Exploratory analyses of tumor response (23%) and 6-month progression-free survival (46%) for the combination in this study were compared with historical control data for single-agent bevacizumab from GOG 229E (response: 13% and 6-month progression-free survival: 40%) (40) and to single-agent temsirolimus in a National Cancer Institute of Canada study (response: 7%). Neither tumor response nor 6-month progression-free survival was statistically significantly higher for the combination than for either single-agent alone.

The epothilones are a new class of nontaxane tubulin polymerization agents obtained by fermentation of the myxobacteria Sorangium cellulosum (41). The chief components of the fermentation process are epothilones A and B. In 1994, the National Cancer Institute discovered that the epothilones possess potent cytotoxic activity. The cytotoxic activities of the epothilones, like those of the taxanes, have been linked to stabilization of the microtubules, which results in mitotic arrest at the G2/M transition (42,43). Importantly, the epothilones are active against various taxane-resistant cell lines, including those with overexpression of multidrug resistance and with mutations in the beta tubulin gene. Ixabepilone (BMS-247550) is a semisynthetic analog of the natural product epothilone B. Ixabepilone is active in both taxane-naive and taxane-pretreated populations.

In GOG study 129P, 50 evaluable women were treated with ixabepilone at 40 mg/m^2 over 3 h every

21 days. The overall response rate was 12%, with one complete and 5 partial responses. This occurred despite 94% of the patients having failed prior paclitaxel (29). Ixabepilone has been successfully combined with carboplatin in a phase I study (44). In vivo testing has shown that ixabepilone may enhance the antitumor effects of antiangiogenic therapy by direct cytotoxicity and also indirectly via the killing of tumor-associated endothelial cells (43,45).

Overall, three novel agents have shown promise in endometrial cancer: bevacizumab, mTor inhibitors (see below), and ixabepilone. The role of these agents in combination with the paclitaxel/carboplatin backbone under study in GOG 209 (bevacizumab and mTor inhibition) or carboplatin (ixabepilone) in the initial therapy of endometrial cancer is not known. GOG 86P is a randomized phase II study that is evaluating these 3 treatments with the paclitaxel/carboplatin arm of GOG 209 serving as a historical reference. GOG 86P intends to eliminate treatments with insufficient activity to warrant further investigation in this patient population. No attempt will be made to compare the arms.

Three mTOR inhibitors, temsirolimus (CCI-779), deforolimus (AP23573, MK-8669), and everolimus (RAD001), are currently in clinical trials in endometrial cancer. Preliminary results of a phase II trial of temsirolimus in recurrent or metastatic endometrial cancer (chemotherapy-naive patients, with up to one prior line of hormonal therapy) demonstrated encouraging results with 5 confirmed partial responses (26%) out of 19 evaluable patients (46). Of note, three of the partial responses were in patients with papillary serous tumors. Evaluation of a second cohort, women who must have had treatment with one prior regimen of cytotoxic chemotherapy, revealed a response rate of 7% (47).

A phase II trial of everolimus at MD Anderson Cancer Center, in patients with one or two prior chemotherapy regimens, reported stable disease ≥8 weeks in 44% of patients and stable disease at ≥20 weeks in 21% (48). Entry was limited to patients with endometrioid histology.

A phase II trial of ridaforolimus (AP23573 and MK-8669, formerly deforolimus) in recurrent or metastatic endometrial cancer and carcinosarcoma of the uterus (up to two prior cytotoxic regimens) has recently completed enrollment. The primary efficacy endpoint was Clinical Benefit Response (CBR), defined as a complete or partial response or prolonged stable disease (16 weeks). Seven of the first 19 patients achieved CBR, allowing expansion to the second stage. Enrollment is now complete. Demographic data are available for 35 (median 66 years; range 46–89) patients who completed treatment: 23 adenocarcinomas, 5 carcinosarcomas, 6 papillary serous carcinomas, and 1 clear cell carcinoma. Thirty-four patients had prior chemotherapy including doxorubicin, taxanes or platinum agents. Fourteen of the 26 patients with available history had prior pelvic RT. Nine of 27 (33%) patients evaluable for response had CBRs, including two partial responses. One CBR was in a patient with papillary serous carcinoma, the other patients achieving CBR, including the partial responders, had adenocarcinomas. Seven patients achieving CBR remain on treatment. The most common adverse events were fatigue (33%), anemia (33%), mouth sores (30%), and nausea/vomiting (30%). AP23573 shows encouraging single-agent activity in pretreated patients with advanced, progressive endometrial cancer and is well tolerated (49).

GOG 248 is a randomized phase II trial of temsirolimus or the combination of hormones (tamoxifen and MA) plus temsirolimus in women with advanced, recurrent or persistent endometrial carcinoma. This trial opened in September 2008 and stage I completed in October 2009. Stage I accrued 43 of a target of 84 patients. As of December 2009, the hormone combination arm was closed to accrual for excess venous thromboses, which included deep venous thrombosis (five patients) and nonfatal pulmonary embolism (two patients), one sudden death, and one myocardial infarction. Eleven of 21 eligible patients had prior chemotherapy. Of seven eligible patients still on study at that time, five continued on the combination, one continued on temsirolimus alone, and one stopped all study therapy. Overall, 3 of 21 eligible patients had a partial response. There were no venous thromboses on the temsirolimus arm, which completed accrual in Novermber 2010 (total enrolled on the temsirolimus arm: 51). The combination of temsirolimus with MA/tamoxifen appears to result in an unacceptable rate of venous thrombosis and its activity is not sufficient to offset its risk of thrombotic events. Single-agent temsirolimus results should be available in the near future (50).

A phase I trial of paclitaxel, carboplatin, and temsirolimus (National Cancer Institute study NCT00408655) in patients with advanced solid malignancies suitable for carboplatin and paclitaxel chemotherapy who had not received more than two prior lines of chemotherapy has been completed. Thirty-one eligible patients have been treated and 27 are evaluable for toxicity. Of the 26 patients with follow-up data, there have been 10 with partial response (38.5%; median duration: 7.1 months) and 12 with stable disease (46%; median duration: 6.9 months). One patient developed progressive disease and three were nonevaluable. The results indicate this combination requires additional assessment in a Phase II setting (51).

Data from a randomized phase II trial of ridaforolimus compared with progestin or chemotherapy in patients with advanced endometrial carcinoma (NCT00739830) has recently been presented. In this trial, the experimental arm was comprised of oral ridaforolimus, while the experimental arm was comprised of the investigators choice of oral MPA tablets daily or oral MA tablets four times per day or chemotherapy (carboplatin, paclitaxel, doxorubicin, pegylated liposomal doxorubicin, or topotecan) administered as a single agent or as a doublet. The chemotherapy was administered at doses and schedules chosen by the investigator. Exclusion criteria included more than two lines of chemotherapy, chemotherapy for recurrent or metastatic disease administered within 6 months of adjuvant therapy, and any prior therapy with hormonal agents. Interim analysis was based on 114 patients. Patients in the trial were randomized to receive either oral ridaforolimus (n = 57), or oral progestin (n = 48) or chemotherapy (n = 9). The interim analysis demonstrated a statistically significant 1.7-month difference in median progression-free survival (ridaforolimus, 3.6 months; standard of care, 1.9 months, p = .007) and an HR of 0.52. The most common adverse events observed with ridaforolimus were mucositis (38.2%), stomatitis (21.8%), and hyperglycemia (27.3%), which have been observed in previous studies and are considered to be class effects of mTOR inhibitors. Overall, patients treated with ridaforolimus had significantly more serious adverse events (23.6%) than patients treated with the standard of care (3.8%) (52).

Endometrial cancer is the most common gynecologic malignancy, and treatment options for patients with advanced/recurrent disease are limited. The optimal adjuvant treatment strategy for these patients is still not well-defined, but much knowledge has been gained regarding more optimal and well-tolerated chemotherapy combinations. Additionally, antivascular agents as well as agents targeting the PI3K/Akt/mTOR pathway show promise in this malignancy.

■ REFERENCES

1. Jemal A, Siegel R, Ward E, et al. Cancer statistics. *CA Cancer J Clin.* 2009;59:225–249.

2. Randall ME, Filiaci VL, Muss H, et al. Randomized Phase III trial of whole-abdominal irradiation versus doxorubicin and cisplatin chemotherapy in advanced endometrial carcinoma: A Gynecologic Oncology Group Study. *J Clin Oncol.* 2006;24(1):36–44.

3. Homesley HD, Filiaci V, Gibbons SK, et al. A randomized phase III trial in advanced endometrial carcinoma of surgery and volume directed radiation followed by cisplatin and doxorubicin with or without paclitaxel: A Gynecologic Oncology Group study. *Gynecol Oncol.* 2009;112(3):543–552.

4. Greven K, Winter K, Underhill K, et al. Final analysis of RTOG 9708: Adjuvant postoperative irradiation combined with cisplatin/paclitaxel chemotherapy following surgery for patients with high-risk endometrial cancer. *Gynecol Oncol.* 2006;103(1):155–159.

5. Ettinger D, Allegra J, Bertino P, et al. Megestrol acetate vs. tamoxifen in advanced breast cancer: Correlation of hormone receptors and response. *Sem Oncol.* 1986;13:9–14.

6. Johnson P, Bonomi P, Kenning M, et al. Megestrol acetate: First-line therapy for advanced breast cancer. *Sem Oncol.* 1988;13:15–19.

7. Mortel R, Zaino R, Satyaswaroop G. Designing a schedule of progestin administration in the control of endometrial carcinoma growth in the nude mouse model. *Am J Obstet Gynecol.* 1990;162:928–936.

8. Carlson J, Allegra J, Day T, et al. Tamoxifen and endometrial carcinoma: Alterations in estrogen and progesterone receptors in untreated patients and combination hormonal therapy in advanced neoplasia. *Am J Obstet Gynecol.* 1984;149:149–153.

9. Mortel R, Levy C, Wolff JP, et al. Female sex steroid receptors in postmenopausal endometrial carcinoma and biochemical response to an antiestrogen. *Cancer Res.* 1986;41:1140–1147.

10. Fiorica M, Brunetto VL, Hanjani P, et al. Phase II trial of alternating course of megestrol acetate and tamoxifen in advanced endometrial carcinoma: A Gynecologic Oncology Group Study. *Gynecol Oncol.* 2004;91:10–14.

11. Lentz SS, Brady MF, Major FJ, et al. High-dose megestrol acetate in advanced or recurrent endometrial carcinoma: A Gynecologic Oncology Group study. *J Clin Oncol.* 1996;14:357–361.

12. Thigpen JT, Brady MF, Alvarez RD, et al. Oral medroxyprogesterone acetate in the treatment of advanced or recurrent endometrial carcinoma: A dose-response study by the Gynecologic Oncology Group. *J Clin Oncol.* 1999;17:1736–1744.

13. Whitney CW, Brunetto VL, Zaino RJ, et al. Phase II study of medroxyprogesterone acetate plus tamoxifen

in advanced endometrial carcinoma: A Gynecologic Oncology Group study. *Gynecol Oncol.* 2004;91:4–9.

14. Thigpen T, Brady MF, Homesley HD, et al. Tamoxifen in the treatment of advanced or recurrent endometrial carcinoma: A Gynecologic Oncology Group Study. *J Clin Oncol.* 2001;19:364–367.

15. Rose, PG, Brunetto VL, VanLe L, et al. A phase II trial of anastrozole in advanced recurrent or persistent endometrial carcinoma: A Gynecologic Oncology Group Study. *Gynecol Oncol.* 2000;78(2):212–216.

16. Thigpen H, Buchsbaum H, Mangan C, et al. Phase II trial of adriamycin in the treatment of advanced or recurrent endometrial carcinoma. *Cancer Treat Rep.* 1979;63:21–27.

17. Thigpen JT, Blessing JA, Homesley H, et al. Phase II trial of cisplatin as first-line chemotherapy in patients with advanced or recurrent endometrial carcinoma: A Gynecologic Oncology Group Study. *Gynecol Oncol.*1989;33:68–70.

18. Long HL, Pfeifle DM, Wieand HS, et al. Phase II evaluation of carboplatin in advanced endometrial carcinoma. *J Natl Cancer Inst.* 1988;80(4):276.

19. Green JB, 3rd, Green S, Alberts DS, et al. Carboplatin therapy in advanced endometrial cancer. *Obstet Gynecol.* 1990;75:696–700.

20. Ball HG, Blessing JA, Lentz SS, et al. A phase II trial of paclitaxel in patients with advanced or recurrent adenocarcinoma of the endometrium: A Gynecologic Oncology Group study. *Gynecol Oncol.* 1996;62:278–281.

21. Sutton GP, Blessing JA, DeMars LR, et al. A phase II Gynecologic Oncology Group trial of ifosfamide and mesna in advanced or recurrent adenocarcinoma of the endometrium. *Gynecol Oncol.* 1996;63:25–27.

22. Wadler S, Levy DE, Lincoln ST, et al. Topotecan is an active agent in the first-line treatment of metastatic or recurrent endometrial carcinoma: Eastern Cooperative Oncology Group Study E3E93. *J Clin Oncol.* 2003;21(11):2110–2114.

23. Homesley HD, Blessing JA, Sorosky J, et al. Phase II trial of liposomal doxorubicin at 40 mg/m(2) every 4 weeks in endometrial carcinoma: A Gynecologic Oncology Group Study. *Gynecol Oncol.* 2005;98(2):294–298.

24. Lincoln S, Blessing JA, Lee RB, et al. Activity of paclitaxel as second-line chemotherapy in endometrial carcinoma: A Gynecologic Oncology Group study. *Gynecol Oncol.* 2003;88:277–281.

25. Muggia FM, Blessing JA, Sorosky J, et al. A Phase II trial of the pegylated liposomal doxorubicin in previously treated metastatic endometrial cancer: A Gynecologic Oncology Group Study. *J Clin Oncol.* 2002;20(9):2360–2364.

26. Miller DS, Blessing JA, Lentz SS, et al. *A Phase II trial of topotecan in patients with advanced, persistent or recurrent endometrial carcinoma: A Gynecologic Oncology Group Study.* Presented at the 37th Annual Meeting of the American Society of Clinical Oncology, San Francisco, CA; May 12–15, 2001.

27. Fracasso PM, Blessing JA, Molpus KL, et al. Phase II study of oxaliplatin as second-line chemotherapy in endometrial carcinoma: A Gynecologic Oncology Group study. *Gynecol Oncol.* 2003;103:523–526.

28. Garcia AA, Blessing JA, Nolte S, et al. A phase II evaluation of weekly docetaxel in the treatment of recurrent or persistent endometrial carcinoma: A study by the Gynecologic Oncology Group. *Gynecol Oncol.* 2008;111:22–26.

29. Don S. Dizon DS, Blessing JA, et al. Phase II trial of ixabepilone as second-line treatment in advanced endometrial cancer: Gynecologic Oncology Group Trial 129-P. *J Clin Oncol.* 2009;27(19):3104–3108.

30. Thigpen JT, Brady MF, Homesley HD, et al. Phase III trial of doxorubicin with or without cisplatin in advanced endometrial carcinoma: A gynecologic oncology group study. *J Clin Oncol.* 2004;22:3902–3908.

31. Fleming GF, Filiaci VL, Bentley RC, et al. Phase III randomized trial of doxorubicin + cisplatin versus doxorubicin + 24-h paclitaxel + filgrastim in endometrial carcinoma: A Gynecologic Oncology Group study. *Ann Oncol.* 2004;15:1173–1178.

32. Fleming GF, Brunetto VL, Cella D, et al. Phase III trial of doxorubicin plus cisplatin with or without paclitaxel plus filgrastim in advanced endometrial carcinoma: A Gynecologic Oncology Group Study. *J Clin Oncol.* 2004;22(11):2159–2166.

33. McMeekin DS, Sill MW, Benbrook D, et al. Gynecologic Oncology Group. A phase II trial of thalidomide in patients with refractory endometrial cancer and correlation with angiogenesis biomarkers: A Gynecologic Oncology Group study. *Gynecol Oncol.* 2007;105(2):508–516.

34. Talvensaari-Mattila A, Soini Y, Santala M, et al. VEGF and its receptors (flt-1 and KDR/flk-1) as prognostic indicators in endometrial carcinoma. *Tumour Biol.* 2005;26(2):81–87.

35. Saito M, Sato Y, Watanabe J, et al. Angiogenic factors in normal endometrium and endometrial adenocarcinoma. *Pathol Int.* 2007;57(3):140–147.

36. Yokoyama Y, Charnock-Jones DS, Licence D, et al. Expression of vascular endothelial growth factor (VEGF)-D and its receptor, VEGF receptor 3, as a prognostic factor in endometrial carcinoma. *Clin Cancer Res.* 2003;9(4):1361–1369.

37. Giatromanolaki A, Sivridis E, Brekken R, et al. The angiogenic "vascular endothelial growth factor/flk-1 (KDR) receptor" pathway in patients with endometrial carcinoma: prognostic and therapeutic implications. *Cancer.* 2001;92(10):2569–2577.

38. Hirai M, Nakagawara A, Oosaki T, et al. Expression of vascular endothelial growth factors (VEGF-A/VEGF-1 and VEGF-C/VEGF-2) in postmenopausal uterine endometrial carcinoma. *Gynecol Oncol.* 2001;80(2):181–188.

39. Giatromanolaki A, Koukourakis MI, Turley H, et al. Tumour and Angiogenesis Research Group. Phosphorylated KDR expression in endometrial cancer cells relates to HIF1alpha/VEGF pathway and unfavorable prognosis. *Mod Pathol.* 2006;19(5):701–707.

40. Aghajanian C, Sill MW, Darcy K, et al. A phase II evaluation of bevacizumab in the treatment of recurrent or persistent endometrial cancer: A Gynecologic Oncology Group (GOG) study [abstract 5531]. *J Clin Oncol.* 2009;27:15s.

41. Gerth K, Bedorf N, Hofle G, et al. Epothilons A and B: Antifungal and cytotoxic compounds from Sorangium cellulosum (Myxobacteria): Production, physico-chemical and biological properties. *J Antibiot (Tokyo).* 1996;49:560–563.

42. Bollag DM, McQueney PA, Zhu J, et al. Epothilones, a new class of microtubule-stabilizing agents with a Taxol-like mechanism of action. *Cancer Res.* 1995;55:2325–2333.

43. Kowalski RJ, Giannakakou P, Hamel E. Activities of the microtubule-stabilizing agents epothilones A and B with purified tubulin and in cells resistant to paclitaxel (Taxol). *J Biol Chem.* 1997;272:2534–2541.

44. Plummer R, Molife R, Verrill M, et al. Phase I and pharmacokinetic study of BMS-247550 in combination with carboplatin in patients with advanced solid malignancies [abstract]. *J Clin Oncol.* 2002;21:2125.

45. Lee FYF, Covello KL, Castaneda S, et al. Synergistic antitumor activity of ixabepilone (BMS- 247550) plus bevacizumab in multiple in vivo tumor models. *Clin Cancer Res.* 2008;14(24):8123–8131.

46. Oza, AM, Elit L, Biagi J, et al. Molecular correlates associated with a phase II study of temsirolimus (CCI-77) in patients with metastatic or recurrent endometrial cancer-NCIC IND 160 [Abstract 3003]. *J Clin Oncol.* 2006;24:18S.

47. Oza, AM, Elit, L, Provencher J, et al. NCIC CTG IND 160b: Phase II study of CCI-779 (temsirolimus) in patients with metastatic and/or locally advanced recurrent endometrial cancer [abstract 5516]. *J Clin Oncol.* 2004;26:15S.

48. Slomovitz BM, Lu KH, Johnston T, et al. A phase II study of oral mammalian target of rapamycin (mTor) inhibitor, RAD001 (everolimus) in patients with recurrent endometrial cancer (EC) [abstract 5502]. *J Clin Oncol.* 2008;26:15S.

49. Colombo N, McMeekin S, Schwartz P, et al. A phase II trial of the mTOR inhibitor AP23573 as a single agent in advanced endometrial cancer [abstract 5516]. *J Clin Oncol.* 2007;25:18S.

50. Fleming GF, Filiaci V, Hanjani P, et al. Hormone therapy plus temsirolimus for endometrial carcinoma (EC): Gynecologic Oncology Group trial #248 [abstract 5014]. *J Clin Oncol.* 2011;29:15S.

51. Oza A, Poveda A, Del Campo JM, et al. *A randomized phase II trial of ridaforolimus compared with progestin or chemotherapy in female adult patients with advanced endometrial carcinoma.* Presented at the 13th Biennial Meeting of the International Gynecologic Cancer Society, Prague, Czech Republic, October 2010.

52. Oza AM, Kollmannsberger C. Phase I study of temsirolimus (CCI-779), carboplatin, and paclitaxel in patients with advanced solid tumors: NCIC GTG IND 179 [abstract 3558]. *J Clin Oncol.* 2009;27:15s.

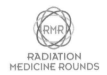

Biologic Agents and Immune Therapy in Gynecologic Cancers

Madeleine Courtney-Brooks and Linda R. Duska*

Division of Gynecologic Oncology, University of Virginia, Charlottesville, VA

■ ABSTRACT

It is estimated that in the United States in 2010, there were more than 83,000 new cases of gynecologic cancer diagnosed and more than 27,000 deaths from gynecologic cancer. Gynecologic malignancies as a group are the third leading cause of cancer-related deaths in women, behind lung and breast cancers. Currently, the mainstay of systemic treatment for gynecologic malignancies is cytotoxic chemotherapy, but new approaches to treatment are needed. Recently developed strategies for the systemic treatment of gynecologic malignancies have centered on inhibiting angiogenesis or targeting oncogenic signal transduction pathways essential to the growth of cancer cells. This chapter provides a summary of biologic, targeted, and immunotherapeutic strategies for the treatment of gynecologic cancers.

Keywords: gynecologic cancers, targeted therapy, antiangiogenesis, monoclonal antibodies, small molecule tyrosine kinase inhibitors, rapamycin analogues, immunotherapy

■ INTRODUCTION

The development of cancer is a complex heterogeneous process. Cancer cell genotypes are the product of changes in cell physiology that together result in malignant growth. These changes include altered production of growth signals, resistance to antigrowth signals, evasion of apoptosis, limitless potential to replicate, sustained angiogenesis, and tissue invasion and metastasis (1). The mainstays of systemic therapy for gynecologic cancers are cytotoxic chemotherapeutic agents. Despite the variety of chemotherapeutic agents available, new tactics for improving the care of women with gynecologic malignancies are needed.

New approaches to treating gynecologic malignancies have focused on inhibiting angiogenesis and targeting the oncogenic signal transduction pathways crucial for the growth of cancer cells. Agents are targeted to alter these signal transduction pathways by blocking an extracellular transmembrane receptor, binding to a serum protein such as vascular endothelial growth factor (VEGF) or by interrupting the actions of intracellular proteins further downstream (2–5). It is assumed that cancer cells are overexpressing various proteins in the signal transduction pathways and are a preferred target for these molecules

*Corresponding author, Department of Obstetrics and Gynecology, Division of Gynecologic Oncology, PO Box 800712, University of Virginia, Charlottesville, VA 22908

E-mail address: lduska@virginia.edu

Radiation Medicine Rounds 2:3 (2011) 401–424.
DOI: 10.5003/2151–4208.2.3.401

compared with normal cells. In theory, this should result in a therapy that is more cancer-cell specific and less toxic for patients. Currently, a number of molecular-targeting strategies are being tested in clinical trials (Table 1) and will be the focus of this review. There are a number of clinical trials involving women with gynecologic malignancies that are currently recruiting patients. A selected list is presented in Table 2. We refer the reader to www.clinicaltrials. gov for a comprehensive list of available trials.

■ ANTIANGIOGENIC AGENTS

Angiogenesis is a physiologic process essential to the survival of both primary and metastatic malignant tumors. It is crucial for supplying a number of substances to tissues including oxygen, nutrients, hormones, and growth factors. It is thought that without angiogenesis, tumor implants would be unable to grow greater than 1 to 2 mm in size (6). There are a number of pathways that contribute to angiogenesis including VEGF, platelet-derived growth factor (PDGF), and fibroblast growth factor (FGF) signaling pathways. Due to the central role of the VEGF-signaling pathway in tumor angiogenesis and growth, it provides one of the most promising targets for therapeutic inhibition (4).

There are two broad classes of anti-VEGF agents which have been developed for clinical use. The first class consists of large molecules, which target VEGF itself and tend to be administered intravenously. The second class consists of small molecules which target tyrosine kinase activity and downstream signaling in the angiogenesis signaling cascade (2).

TABLE 1   Selected targeted therapies in gynecologic cancers

Targeted Pathway	Drug	Chemistry	Main Molecular Targets
Angiogenesis	Bevacizumab	Humanized monoclonal antibody	VEGF-A
	Aflibercept	Soluble fusion protein	VEGF-A ligand
	Sunitinib	TKI	VEGFR, PDGFR
	Pazopanib	TKI	VEGFR 1–3, PDGFR, c-KIT
	Brivanib	TKI	VEGFR2, FGFR 1 and 2
	Cediranib	TKI	VEGFR 1–3, c-KIT
	Valatanib	TKI	VEGFR 1–3
	Vargatef	TKI	VEGFR, PDGFR, FGFR
EGFR	Cetuximab	Chimerized monoclonal antibody	EGFR
	Trastuzumab	Humanized monoclonal antibody	HER2
	Erlotinib	TKI	EGFR ATP binding domain
	Gefitinib	TKI	EGFR ATP binding domain
	Lapatinib	TKI	EGFR, HER 2 intracellular tyrosine kinase domains
Multiple kinases	Imatinib	TKI	Abl, c-KIT, PDGFR
	Sorafenib	Multitargeted kinase inhibitor	Raf/MEK/ERK pathway, VEGFR, PDGFR-β
	Dasatinib	Multitargeted kinase inhibitor	Src, PDGFR, c-KIT
	Vandetanib	Multitargeted kinase inhibitor	VEGFR2, EGFR
PI3-kinase/Akt/ mTOR	Temsirolimus	Rapamycin analog	mTOR
	Deforolimus	Rapamycin analog	mTOR
	Everolimus	Rapamycin analog	mTOR
	Perifosine (KRX-0401)	Alkylphospholipid	Akt, PI3K
	SF1126	RGDS-conjugated LY294002 prodrug	mTOR/PI3K
	PX886	Wortmannin derivative	PI3K-α, β
	GDC-0941	Thieno[3,2-d]pyrimidine derivative	PI3K

VEGF, vascular endothelial growth factor; VEGFR, vascular endothelial growth factor receptor; PDGFR, platelet-derived endothelial cell growth factor receptor; FGFR, fibroblast growth factor receptor; EGFR, epidermal growth factor receptor; HER2, human epidermal growth factor; mTOR, mammalian target of rapamycin; PI3K, phosphotidylinositol-3-kinase.

Bevacizumab

Bevacizumab is a humanized immunoglobulin (Ig) G1 monoclonal antibody directed against VEGF-A (7). Several phase III clinical trials investigating bevacizumab have demonstrated improved survival in metastatic colon cancer (8–10), metastatic breast cancer (11–13), and non–small cell lung cancer (14–16). It is currently approved by the Food and Drug Administration (FDA) in combination with chemotherapy for the treatment of several advanced malignancies, including colorectal cancer, renal cell carcinoma, glioblastoma, and non–small cell lung cancer. Bevacizumab was previously approved for the treatment of breast cancer but the FDA has recently recommended withdrawing the indication (17).

In epithelial ovarian cancer (EOC), several phase II trials have shown activity of bevacizumab in patients with recurrent disease. A study by Burger et al. conducted by the Gynecologic Oncology Group (GOG) evaluated the efficacy of bevacizumab as single-agent therapy in women with EOC or primary peritoneal cancer (PPC) who had persistent or recurrent disease after receiving one or two prior cytotoxic regimens (18). In this study population, 21% of patients had a clinical response and 40% had a progression-free survival (PFS) period of at least 6 months. Median PFS was 4.7 months and median overall survival (OS) was 17 months. A second study conducted by Cannistra et al. (19) investigated the efficacy of bevacizumab as single-agent therapy for women with platinum-resistant EOC or PPC who experienced disease progression during or within 3 months of discontinuing topotecan or liposomal doxorubicin and had received no more than three prior treatment regimens. In this heavily pretreated population, a partial clinical response was seen in 16% of patients; median PFS and OS were 4.4 and 10.7 months, respectively. However, this trial was closed early due to a high proportion of patients experiencing gastrointestinal perforations (11%). Based on the promising results of phase II trials, bevacizumab was included in the treatment schema of two front-line placebo-controlled phase III trials to determine whether its addition to standard chemotherapy would result in an improvement in survival.

The first of these phase III trials was initiated by the GOG and preliminary results have been recently presented (20). Eligible women had stage III or stage IV EOC, PPC, or fallopian tube cancer (FTC) and had undergone surgical staging. Participants were randomized to one of three arms: (1) CT (intravenous

[i.v.] carboplatin area under the curve (AUC) of 6 plus paclitaxel 175 mg/m^2 for cycles 1–6) + placebo cycles 2–22; (2) CT plus concurrent bevacizumab (15 mg/kg) cycles 2–6 + placebo cycles 7–22; or (3) CT + concurrent bevacizumab cycles 2–6 + maintenance bevacizumab cycles 7–22. The hazard ratio of first progression or death for arm 3 relative to arm 1 was 0.717 (95% CI: 0.625–0.824, $p < .0001$), demonstrating that front-line treatment of EOC, PPC, and FTC with carboplatin and paclitaxel plus concurrent and maintenance bevacizumab prolongs PFS. However, the improvement in PFS was modest (3.8 months) and the impact of bevacizumab on OS is not known.

A second phase III trial was conducted by the Gynecologic Cancer InterGroup (ICON 7). Eligible women included those with stage I–IIA ovarian cancer if high risk (grade 3 or clear cell histology) and all women with stage IIB–IV disease that had surgical debulking with the aim of maximal surgical cytoreduction. Patients were randomized to either (a) i.v. carboplatin AUC of 6 plus paclitaxel 175 mg/m^2 for cycles 1–6 or (b) i.v. carboplatin AUC of 6 plus paclitaxel 175 mg/m^2 for cycles 1–6 and concurrent bevacizumab (7.5 mg/kg) cycles 2–18. Initial results were presented at the European Society for Medical Oncology (ESMO) conference in 2010 (21). The addition of concurrent and maintenance bevacizumab to standard chemotherapy statistically improved PFS. Long-term results for PFS and OS are expected next year.

Also recently presented are the results of the OCEANS trial, a randomized, double-blinded, placebo-controlled phase III trial of carboplatin and gemcitabine with or without bevacizumab in patients with platinum-sensitive, recurrent EOC, FTC, or PPC (22). The trial enrolled 484 patients and had a median follow-up of 24 months. Patients receiving bevacizumab in conjunction with carboplatin and gemcitabine for six cycles followed by single-agent bevacizumab until disease progression had an increased PFS (HR = 0.484, $p < .0001$) and an increase of 21% in the objective response rate ($p < .0001$) compared with patients who received only carboplatin and gemcitabine.

Although bevacizumab has generally been well tolerated, there are several potentially serious side effects associated with its administration. Gastrointestinal perforation is a known complication of bevacizumab therapy and has resulted in the closure of a phase II trial in recurrent ovarian cancer (19). The actual rate of bowel perforation among ovarian cancer patients varies in the literature. Based on the results of case series and phase II trials, the rate of bowel perforations is estimated to be 5.4% (23). Preliminary results of phase III trials demonstrated rates of 1% to 2% (20,21). Completion of phase III trials should give a better estimate of the rate of bowel perforation among bevacizumab-treated patients, particularly those who have not been heavily pretreated.

Other potential complications of bevacizumab therapy include hypertension (both newly diagnosed and worsening severity of pre-existing disease), proteinuria, arterial thromboembolism and hemorrhage, reversible posterior leukoencephalopathy syndrome (RPLS), wound healing complications and fistula (24,25).

Aflibercept

Aflibercept, also known as VEGF-Trap, is a soluble fusion protein consisting of truncated VEGFR1 and VEGFR2 binding domains combined with the Fc portion of IgG1. Functioning as a decoy receptor, it binds with high affinity to the VEGF-A ligand and prevents VEGF1 and VEGF2 binding and stimulation (26). Ovarian cancer mouse models have demonstrated that the administration of aflibercept results in the inhibition of both ascites and tumor burden (27). Published phase II studies performed in patients with platinum-resistant lung adenocarcinoma (28) and recurrent or metastatic urothelial cancer (29), demonstrate that it is well tolerated, but has minimal single-agent activity.

A phase II trial of aflibercept in patients with recurrent, platinum-resistant EOC has recently been presented (30). This was a randomized, double-blind, multicenter, two-stage trial of single-agent aflibercept administered intravenously every 2 weeks. In this heavily pretreated population, 11% experienced a partial response (PR). A second phase II trial of aflibercept in combination with docetaxel in recurrent EOC, FTC, or PPC was also recently presented (31). A total of 49 patients were enrolled. The objective response rate was 54%, including 10 complete responders. Median PFS and OS were 6.2 and 24.3 months, respectively. Currently there is an active, but not recruiting phase I/II trial evaluating the use of aflibercept in combination with liposomal doxorubicin for the treatment of persistent/recurrent

EOC and phase II trials investigating its use as a single agent in the treatment of persistent/recurrent endometrial cancer and locally advanced, unresectable or metastatic leiomyosarcoma or carcinosarcoma.

Sunitinib

Sunitinib is an orally available tyrosine kinase inhibitor (TKI), which has a high binding affinity for VEGFR and PDGFR (32). It has been FDA approved for the treatment of gastrointestinal tumors resistant to or intolerant of treatment with imitanib, advanced renal cell carcinoma, and, most recently, locally advanced or metastatic pancreatic neuroendocrine tumors. The GOG conducted a phase II study to determine its activity as a second- or third-line agent among women with recurrent uterine leiomyosarcoma (33). Unfortunately, of the 23 patients enrolled, only 2 (8.7%) achieved a PR and 4 (17.4%) maintained PFS at 6 months. Median PFS was only 1.5 months. Thus, it does not appear to be an agent which results in a significant response rate or disease stabilization among women with recurrent uterine leiomyosarcoma. A recently presented phase II study suggests that sunitinib has tolerability and activity in women with advanced ovarian and endometrial cancer (34–37). There are currently a number of phase II trials investigating its use in recurrent or persistent EOC, PPC, or FTC, as well as a GOG-sponsored trial in recurrent clear cell cancer of the ovary.

Pazopanib

Pazopanib is an oral TKI which primarily inhibits VEGFR1, VEGFR2, and VEGFR3, as well as PDGFR and c-KIT (38). It is now FDA approved for the treatment of advanced renal cell carcinoma. A recent phase II study investigated the use of pazopanib in recurrent EOC, FTC, or PPC as defined by a new elevation of CA-125 (39). In this population, 31% of patients had a CA-125 response. The treatment was generally well tolerated and the most common adverse events leading to study drug discontinuation were an elevation in ALT (8%) or AST (8%).

The use of pazopanib has also been investigated in advanced/recurrent cervical cancer. Recently, results of a randomized phase IIB trial examining the effects of pazopanib or lapatinib, another TKI that

TABLE 2 Active, recruiting clinical trials involving biologic therapies

Class	Drug	Intervention	Study Phase	Patient Population	Protocol ID
Angiogenesis inhibitors	Bevacizumab	1. IV carbo, paclitaxel, bev → bev 2. IV paclitaxel, bev + IP carbo → bev 3. IV paclitaxel, bev + IP cis, paclitaxel → bev	III	Adjuvant and consolidation therapy in stage II–IV EOC, PPC, or FTC	NCT00951496 GOG 252
	Bevacizumab	+/– secondary cytoreduction 1. Carbo, paclitaxel 2. Carbo, paclitaxel, bev	III	Recurrent platinum-sensitive EOC, PPC, or FTC	NCT00565851 GOG 213
	Bevacizumab	1. Carbo, paclitaxel 2. Oxaliplatin, capecitabine 3. Carbo, paclitaxel, bev → bev 4. Oxaliplatin, capecitabine, bev → bev	III	Adjuvant and consolidation therapy in stage II–IV or recurrent stage I EOC or FTC	NCT01081262 GOG 241
	Bevacizumab	1. Paclitaxel or topotecan or liposomal doxorubicin 2. Paclitaxel or topotecan or liposomal doxorubicin + bev	III	Recurrent platinum-resistant EOC, PPC, or FTC	NCT00976911
	Bevacizumab	1. Carbo, paclitaxel 2. Carbo, weekly paclitaxel *optional concurrent and maintenance bev with each arm	III	Adjuvant and consolidation therapy in suboptimal stage III and IV EOC, PPC, or FTC	NCT01167712 GOG 262
	Bevacizumab	1. Cisplatin, paclitaxel 2. Cisplatin, paclitaxel, bev 3. Paclitaxel, topotecan 4. Paclitaxel, topotecan, bev	III	Primary stage IVB, recurrent, or persistent carcinoma of the cervix	NCT00803062 GOG 240
	Bevacizumab	1. Gemcitabine, docetaxel 2. Gemcitabine, docetaxel, bev	III	Recurrent or advanced leiomyosarcoma of the uterus	NCT01012297 GOG 250
	Bevacizumab Everolimus	Bev + everolimus	II	Recurrent EOC, PPC, or FTC	NCT01031381
	Bevacizumab	Gemcitabine, bev	II	Recurrent platinum-resistant EOC, PPC, or FTC	NCT01131039
	Bevacizumab	Carbo, bev, weekly paclitaxel	II	Adjuvant therapy in stage III and IV EOC, PPC, or FTC	NCT01097746
	Bevacizumab	1. Bev 2. Bev, fosbretabulin tromethamine IV	II	Recurrent EOC, PPC, or FTC	NCT01305213 GOG 1861

Continued

405

TABLE 2 *Continued*

Class	Drug	Intervention	Study Phase	Patient Population	Protocol ID
Angiogenesis inhibitors	Bevacizumab Temsirolimus	Bev, temsirolimus	II	Locally advanced, recurrent, metastatic, or progressive EOC, endometrial cancer, liver cancer, islet cell cancer, or carcinoid tumor	NCT01101126
	Bevacizumab	Bev, irinotecan	II	Recurrent EOC, PPC, or FTC	NCT01091259
	Bevacizumab	Bev, pegylated liposomal doxorubicin	II	Recurrent platinum-resistant EOC	NCT00945139
	Bevacizumab	Carbo, bev	II	Recurrent platinum-resistant EOC, PPC, or FTC	NCT00744718
	Bevacizumab	Docetaxel, bev	II	Recurrent EOC, PPC, or FTC	NCT00504257
	Bevacizumab Sorafenib	Sorafenib, bevacizumab	II	Recurrent/refractory EOC, FTC, or PPC	NCT00436215
	Bevacizumab Temsirolimus	1. Carbo, paclitaxel, bev 2. Carbo, paclitaxel, temsirolimus 3. Carbo, paclitaxel, ixabepilone	II	Stage III, IVA-B, or recurrent endometrial carcinoma	NCT00977574 GOG 86P
	Bevacizumab	IMRT + cisplatin, bev → carbo, paclitaxel	II	High-risk endometrial carcinoma	NCT01005329
	Bevacizumab	Lenalidomide, liposomal doxorubicin, bev	I	Recurrent, platinum-resistant EOC, PPC or FTC	NCT01202890
	Bevacizumab	Carbo, bev, weekly paclitaxel	I	Neoadjuvant therapy for stage III and IV EOC, PPC, or FTC	NCT01219777
	Bevacizumab	Carbo, paclitaxel, bev, ABT 888	I	Adjuvant therapy in stage II-IV EOC, PPC, or FTC	NCT00989651 GOG 9923
	Bevacizumab	Bev, OC-DC vaccine, cyclophosphamide, fludarabine, ex vivo CD3/CD28-costimulated vaccine-primed peripheral blood autologous T cells	I	Recurrent EOC, PPC or FTC previously vaccinated with autologous tumor vaccine	NCT01312376
	Bevacizumab	IV paclitaxel weekly + IV bev + IP carbo	I	Adjuvant therapy in stage II-IV EOC, PPC, or FTC	NCT01220154
	Bevacizumab	Bev, polyvalent vaccine-KLH conjugate, OPT-821	I	Histologically confirmed EOC, PPC, or FTC	NCT01223235
	Bevacizumab	Carbo, paclitaxel, bev	0	Neoadjuvant therapy for Stage III or IV EOC, PPC, or FTC	NCT01146795
	Sunitinib	Sunitinib	II	Persistent or recurrent clear cell ovarian cancer	NCT00779992 GOG 254
	Sunitinib	Sunitinib	II	Persistent or recurrent EOC, FTC, PPC	NCT00388037

Category	Drug	Regimen	Indication	Phase	NCT
Angiogenesis inhibitors	Sunitinib	Sunitinib	Persistent or recurrent EOC, FTC, PPC	II	NCT00768144
	Pazopanib	1. Pazopanib 2. Placebo	Stage II-IV EOC, FTC or PPC, who have not progressed after first-line chemo	III	NCT00866697
	Pazopanib	Pazopanib	Recurrent platinum-resistant EOC	II	NCT01262014
	Pazopanib	Pazopanib, liposomal doxorubicin	Recurrent stage II-IV EOC, FTC, or PPC	I/II	NCT01035658
	Pazopanib	Pazopanib, oral cyclophosphamide	Platinum-resistant or refractory EOC, FTC, or PPC	I/II	NCT01238770
	Pazopanib	Pazopanib	Recurrent or persistent carcinosarcoma of the uterus	II	NCT01247571 GOG 230D
	Pazopanib	Pazopanib, oral metronomic topotecan	Recurrent or persistent gynecologic tumor	I	NCT00800345
	Brivanib	Brivanib	Recurrent or persistent endometrial cancer	II	NCT00888173 GOG 229I
	Brivanib	Brivanib	Recurrent or persistent cervical cancer	II	NCT01267253 GOG 227G
	Cediranib	1. Carbo, paclitaxel, placebo → placebo 2. Carbo, paclitaxel, cediranib → placebo 3. Carbo, paclitaxel, cediranib → cediranib	Platinum-sensitive, relapsed EOC, FTC, or PPC	II/III	NCT00532194 ICON 6
	Cediranib, Olaparib	Cediranib, olaparib	Recurrent pap serous EOC, FTC, or PPC	I/II	NCT01116648
	Cediranib, Olaparib	Cediranib, olaparib	Recurrent EOC, FTC, or PPC	I/II	NCT01115829
	Cediranib	1.Carbo, paclitaxel, placebo 2. Carbo, paclitaxel, cediranib	Unresectable metastatic or recurrent cervical cancer	II	NCT01229930
	Vargatef	1. Carbo, paclitaxel, placebo 2. Carbo, paclitaxel, Vargatef	Adjuvant therapy for Stage IIB-IV EOC, FTC, or PPC	III	NCT01015118
	Vargatef	Vargatef	Recurrent or persistent endometrial cancer	II	NCT01225887 GOG 229K
	Vargatef	Carbo, pegylated liposomal doxorubicin, vargatef	Recurrent, platinum-sensitive EOC, FTC, or PPC	I	NCT01329549 NCT01314105
EGFR inhibitors	Cetuximab	Cetuximab, cisplatin, radiation therapy	Stage IB2-IVB cervical cancer	II	NCT00292955
	Cetuximab	1. Cisplatin, radiation therapy 2. Cisplatin, radiation therapy, cetuximab	Stage IB, II or, IIIB cervical cancer	II	NCT00957411
	Cetuximab	1. Carbo, paclitaxel, cetuximab 2. Carbo, paclitaxel, placebo	Advanced/metastatic cervical cancer	II	NCT00997009
	Cetuximab	Cisplatin, radiation therapy, cetuximab	Stage IB-IVA cervical cancer	I	NCT00104910 GOG 9918
	Trastuzumab	1. Carbo, paclitaxel 2. Carbo, paclitaxel, trastuzumab	Stage III-IV or recurrent UPSC	II	NCT01367002
	Erlotinib	Topotecan, erlotinib	Pretreated, recurrent EOC	II	NCT01003938

Continued

TABLE 2 *Continued*

Class	Drug	Intervention	Study Phase	Patient Population	Protocol ID
Multitargeted tyrosine kinase inhibitors	Sorafenib	1. Carbo, paclitaxel, sorafenib 2. Carbo, paclitaxel	II	Adjuvant therapy for Stage III or IV EOC	NCT00390611
	Sorafenib	Sorafenib, topotecan	II	Platinum-resistant/refractory EOC, FTC, or PPC	NCT01047891
	Sorafenib	Sorafenib, cisplatin, radiation therapy	I/II	Initial treatment for cervical cancer	NCT00510250
	Dasatinib	Dasatinib, carbo, paclitaxel	I	Recurrent or persistent EOC, FTC, or PPC	NCT00672295
	Vandetanib	1. Docetaxel 2. Docetaxel, vandetanib	II	Recurrent EOC, PPC, or FTC	NCT00872989
PI3K/Akt/mTOR inhibitors	Temsirolimus	Carbo, paclitaxel, temsirolimus → temsirolimus	II	Adjuvant and consolidative therapy for Stage III-IV clear cell ovarian carcinoma	NCT01196429 GOG 268
	Temsirolimus	Temsirolimus	II	Recurrent uterine carcinosarcoma	NCT01061606
	Temsirolimus	Temsirolimus	II	Recurrent EOC, PPC or FTC	NCT00926107
	Temsirolimus	Temsirolimus	II	Recurrent, unresectable, or metastatic cervical carcinoma	NCT01026792
	Temsirolimus	Pegylated liposomal doxorubicin, temsirolimus	I	Advanced, refractory endometrial or ovarian cancer	NCT00982631
	Deforolimus	Carbo, paclitaxel, deforolimus	I	Locally advanced or metastatic endometrial, ovarian or solid tumor	NCT01256268
PI3K/Akt/mTOR inhibitors	Everolimus	Letrozole, everolimus	II	Progressive or recurrent endometrial cancer	NCT01068249
	Everolimus	Weekly everolimus, oral topotecan	I	Progressive or recurrent endometrial cancer	NCT00703807
	Everolimus	Carbo, pegylated liposomal doxorubicin, everolimus	I	Recurrent platinum-sensitive EPC, PPC, or FTC in first relapse	NCT01281514
	Everolimus	Cisplatin, radiation therapy, everolimus	I	Primary therapy for stages IIB-IIIB cervical cancer	NCT01217177
	Perifosine	Docetaxel, perifosine	I	Recurrent platinum-resistant EOC, PPC, or FTC	NCT00431054
Aurora kinase inhibitors	MLN 8237	1. Paclitaxel, MLN 8237 2. Paclitaxel	I/II	Recurrent EOC, PPC, or FTC	NCT01091428
PARP inhibitors	Olaparib	1. Carbo, paclitaxel, olaparib 2. Carbo, paclitaxel	II	Recurrent EOC	NCT01081951
	Olaparib	Carbo, olaparib	I	BRCA1/BRCA2-associated, hereditary, or triple negative metastatic or unresectable breast or EOC	NCT00647062
Folate receptor α	Farletuzumab	1. Carbo, taxane, farletuzumab 2. Carbo, taxane, farletuzumab 3. Carbo, taxane	III	Platinum-sensitive EOC, PPC, or FTC in first relapse	NCT00849667
	Farletuzumab	1. Paclitaxel, farletuzumab 2. Paclitaxel	II	Platinum-resistant/refractory recurrent EOC	NCT00738699

Bev, bevacizumab; Carbo, carboplatin.

targets epidermal growth factor receptor (EGFR) and HER2/neu, compared with pazopanib plus lapatinib among women with measureable stage IVB persistent/recurrent cervical cancer was published (40). A total of 228 women were enrolled. At the time of interim analysis, the futility boundary had been crossed for combination therapy compared with lapatinib therapy and the combination arm was discontinued at that time. Overall, 9% of patients in the pazopanib arm responded. Both PFS and OS were longer in the pazopanib arm compared with the lapatinib arm (18.1 vs. 17.1 weeks and 50.7 vs. 39.7 weeks, respectively). A total of 19% of patients in the pazopanib arm discontinued therapy secondary to adverse events, the most common of which were small bowel obstruction (3%) and genital fistula (3%). This suggests that the anti-angiogenesis approach may be superior to EGFR inhibition in this patient population.

Currently there are a number of clinical trials in progress investigating the use of pazopanib in women with ovarian cancer after response to initial therapy as well as among women with advanced or recurrent disease in combination with other agents.

Brivanib

Brivanib is an orally available, selective TKI that primarily targets VEGFR-2, FGFR-1 and FGFR-2 (41). Several phase I studies have demonstrated that brivanib has an acceptable toxicity profile, the most common side effects being transaminase elevations, nausea, and fever, and promising antitumor activity (42,43). Currently there are two GOG-sponsored phase II trials investigating the use of brivanib in recurrent or persistent endometrial and cervical cancer.

Other TKI

Cediranib, valatanib (PTK787/ZK222584), and vargatef (BIBF 1120) are three additional orally available TKIs. Cediranib inhibits VEGFR1, VEGFR2, VEGFR3, and c-KIT (44), valatanib effectively inhibits all three VEGFR tyrosine kinases (45) and vargatef targets all three receptor classes involved in the formation of blood vessels, VEGFR, PDGFR, and FGFR (46). There have been a number of phase I and II trials investigating the use of these agents in gynecologic malignancies, both as single agents and in combination with cytotoxic chemotherapy (47–51).

■ EGFR INHIBITORS

A second molecular pathway which affects cancer evolution and thus is an attractive candidate for targeted therapies is the epidermal growth factor family of tyrosine kinase receptors, known as the ErbB receptors. Four ErbB members have been identified: ErbB1 (also known as EGFR and HER1), ErbB2 (also known as HER2 or Neu), ErbB3 (also known as HER3), and ErbB4 (also known as HER4) (52). The EGFR pathway contributes to a number of processes which are vital to cancer development and progression including cell proliferation, apoptosis, angiogenesis and metastatic spread (53). EGFRs have an extracellular ligand-binding domain, transmembrane domains and intracellular tyrosine kinase domains (54). HER3 lacks tyrosine kinase activity and HER2 does not have a ligand that has been identified. HER2 forms heterodimers with other types of EGFRs, and this heterodimer formation results in altered signal transduction upon ligand binding (55).

Several therapeutic strategies have been developed to target the EGFR family. The strategies which have entered clinical trials include the development of small molecule inhibitors of the receptor tyrosine kinase domain and monoclonal antibodies against the extracellular domain. The best-studied agents and the clinical evidence supporting their use in the treatment of gynecologic cancers are discussed below.

Monoclonal Antibody Inhibitors to EGFR

Cetuximab
Cetuximab is a human/murine chimeric monoclonal antibody that binds with high affinity to the EGFR, competing with EGF and TGF-α binding, thus inhibiting subsequent receptor activation and signaling (56). Cetuximab is currently FDA approved for the treatment of squamous cell cancers of the head and neck, as well as metastatic colorectal cancer.

A phase II trial of single-agent cetuximab in persistent or recurrent EOC or PPC was conducted (57).

A total of 25 patients were enrolled and 22 were evaluable for response. However, the trial was stopped after the first stage due to futility, as only one patient had an objective response. The most common side effect was an acneiform rash, which was present to some degree in 24/25 (96%) of patients. There have also been several phase II trials of cetuximab in combination with other agents for the treatment of EOC. One assessed its use in combination with carboplatin and paclitaxel as initial treatment of advanced stage EOC/FTC/PPC (58). While the vast majority of patients did develop an acneiform rash, overall the combination was adequately tolerated. However, median PFS was only 14.4 months, which was not a prolongation compared with historical data. Finally, GOG 146P was a phase II trial examining the use of cetuximab in combination with carboplatin in women with recurrent platinum-sensitive EOC/PPC whose tumor specimens were EGFR positive (59). Of evaluable patients, 9 of 26 (34%) experienced an objective response and 8 (31%) had stable disease. Nevertheless, this did not meet the preset criteria for opening a second stage.

Recently, the role of cetuximab in advanced cervical cancer has also been examined. GOG 76-DD evaluated the efficacy of concurrent cisplatin and cetuximab in women with advanced, persistent, or recurrent cervical cancer (60). Patients received cisplatin 30 mg/m^2 on days 1 and 8 every 21 days and cetuximab on days 1, 8, and 15. Overall, 69 patients were accrued and eligible for analysis. The objective clinical response rate was 11%. While the regimen was adequately tolerated, it does not appear to have benefit beyond that of cisplatin alone. GOG 9918 was recently presented and was designed to assess the safety of concurrent chemoradiation with cetuximab in locally advanced cervical cancer (61). For women receiving only pelvic irradiation, the combination was fairly well tolerated. For those receiving extended field irradiation, high rates of gastrointestinal and metabolic toxicity were observed. There are a number of phase I and II trials currently in progress evaluating the use of cetuximab with other combinations of agents.

Trastuzumab

A humanized monoclonal antibody against the HER2 receptor that blocks ligand activation, trastuzumab is currently FDA approved for the treatment of HER2/*neu* positive breast cancer as well as gastric and gastroesophageal cancers. Due to promising results in breast cancer, the GOG began a phase II, single-agent trial of trastuzumab in recurrent or refractory EOC or PPC with overexpression of HER2 (62). A total of 837 women were screened, but only 95 tumors (11.4%) exhibited 2+ or 3+ immunohistochemical (IHC) expression of HER2. Ultimately, a total of 45 patients were registered in two stages, with 41 eligible for assessment. Treatment with trastuzumab was well tolerated, but unfortunately the overall objective response rate was only 7.3%. A recently published phase II study in advanced or recurrent HER2 positive endometrial cancer using single-agent trastuzumab therapy also had a similarly low response rate (63). Moreover, trastuzumab as a single agent did not demonstrate activity against endometrial carcinomas with HER2 overexpression. A phase II trial examining the use of trastuzumab in conjunction with carboplatin and paclitaxel in HER2+ patients with advanced or recurrent uterine papillary serous carcinoma is slated to begin recruitment shortly.

Small Molecule Inhibitors

Erlotinib

An orally available, small molecule tyrosine kinase inhibitor, erlotinib is approved for the treatment of non–small cell lung cancer and pancreatic cancer. The most common side effects are skin rash and diarrhea (64). A single-arm phase II study of single-agent erlotinib in recurrent HER1/EGFR positive epithelial ovarian tumors demonstrated that it was generally well tolerated and had a 6% objective response rate (65). Since then, there have been a variety of phase I and phase II trials investigating its use in combination with other agents for the treatment of recurrent EOC (66–69). A phase II study by Hirte et al. (68) demonstrated that erlotinib in combination with carboplatin may be active in patients with platinum-sensitive disease. However, it does not appear to improve response rates when combined with carboplatin and paclitaxel as first line therapy of stage III-IV EOC/FTC/PPC (70). A phase II trial in recurrent cervical squamous cell carcinoma indicates that erlotinib is inactive as a single agent (71).

Gefitinib

Another orally available, small molecule TKI, gefitinib is currently approved for use in non–small cell lung cancer. GOG 170C was a phase II trial evaluating the efficacy of gefitinib in relapsed or persistent EOC or PPC (72). Overall gefitinib was well tolerated, with the most common grade 3 toxicities being skin rash or diarrhea. Only 1 of 27 (3.7%) patients had a clinical response; however, this patient had a mutation in tumor's EGFR, suggesting that prescreening patients for activating mutations in EGFR may improve response rates. A phase II study of gefitinib given in combination with carboplatin and paclitaxel as second-line therapy for EOC/FTC/PPC was recently published (73). A total of 68 women were enrolled, with 60 evaluable for response. An objective tumor response was seen in 31 patients (46%) and the median duration of response was 6.3 and 7.6 months in platinum-resistant/refractory and -sensitive patients, respectively. The most common adverse events were diarrhea, nausea, and neutropenia.

Phase II studies of single-agent gefitinib in recurrent advanced or metastatic cervical and endometrial cancer have shown a general tolerability of the drug, but lack of significant efficacy (74,75).

Lapatinib

Lapatinib is an orally active dual inhibitor of the EGFR and HER2 tyrosine kinases and is approved for use in combination with other therapies in patients with advanced or metastatic HER2 positive breast cancer (76). Several phase I studies of lapatinib have been conducted in gynecologic malignancies. A study by Kimball et al. (77) examined the use of lapatinib in combination with carboplatin in women with platinum-sensitive recurrent ovarian cancer. No dose limiting toxicity was noted. However, several women experienced grade 3 and 4 thrombocytopenia and/or neutropenia, resulting in excessive treatment delays and the early closing of the trial. A second phase I study examined the use of lapatinib in combination with carboplatin and paclitaxel in women with stage III or IV recurrent ovarian cancer (78). In this heavily pretreated population, 10 of 25 (40%) patients experienced grade 3 toxicities, primarily bone marrow suppression. Twenty-one percent of patients achieved a complete response (CR) and 29% had a PR. This study demonstrated that the combination of lapatinib with carboplatin and paclitaxel is well tolerated and also highly active in this patient population. Most recently, the combination of lapatinib and topotecan was evaluated in a phase II trial of platinum-refractory/resistant EOC and PPC (79). The trial was stopped after the first stage due to insufficient activity.

Multitargeted TKIs

Imatinib

Imatinib mesylate is a TKI which has activity against a number of targets including abl, c-kit, and PDGFR (80). It is currently approved for use in a variety of leukemias and myeloproliferative disorders, among other illnesses. Preclinical work indicated that ovarian serous carcinomas commonly express at least one of the targets of imatinib, which led to clinical trials evaluating its use in patients with EOC (81). Multiple phase II trials of imatinib as a single agent for recurrent or persistent EOC/PPC in both platinum-sensitive and platinum-resistant patients have been conducted (82–85). Although imatinib was well tolerated, it demonstrated minimal single-agent activity. A phase II trial investigating its use in combination with docetaxel also resulted in few patients with sustained responses or stable disease (86).

Preclinical studies have also suggested a potential role of the PDGFR system in the pathogenesis of cervical cancer and that cervical cancer cell lines are inhibited by imatinib (87). Unfortunately, a phase II trial of imatinib as single-agent therapy for recurrent or metastatic cervical cancer expressing PDGFR-α demonstrated lack of activity (88).

Sorafenib

An oral multitargeted kinase inhibitor which targets the Raf/MEK/ERK signaling pathway, sorafenib is a potent inhibitor of the VEGFR and PDGFR-β tyrosine kinases (89). It is currently approved for the treatment of unresectable hepatocellular carcinoma, as well as advanced renal cell carcinoma. GOG 170F was conducted to determine its activity and tolerability in patients with recurrent EOC (90). In this patient population, 2 of 59 women (3.4%) achieved a PR, with 12 (20%) demonstrating no progression for at least 6 months. The most common grade ≥3 toxicities were skin manifestations and metabolic disturbances. Sorafenib has also been used in combination with other cytotoxic agents for the treatment of recurrent EOC with acceptable levels of toxicity (34,91). Currently, there are a number of clinical trials underway examining its use in combination with other therapies for the treatment of recurrent EOC, for the initial treatment of cervical cancer in conjunction with radiation and chemosensitization, and as first-line treatment in stage III/IV EOC (92).

Dasatinib

Dasatinib is an oral, multitargeted kinase inhibitor whose targets include SRC, PDGFR, and c-KIT and potently inhibits BCR-ABL (93). It is currently FDA approved for the treatment of chronic myelogenous leukemia (CML) and Philadelphia chromosome-positive acute lymphoblastic leukemia (ALL). Studies have also been initiated in several solid tumors. These early studies indicate that dasatinib is fairly well tolerated, with reported rates of dose-limiting toxicities less than those seen in the treatment of hematologic malignancies (93,94). A phase II trial initiated by the GOG investigating the use of dasatinib in the treatment of recurrent or persistent EOC, FTC, or PPC was closed after the first stage, but results are not yet available. Currently there is a phase I trial open examining its use in combination with carboplatin and paclitaxel in a similar patient population.

Vandetanib

Vandetanib is an orally available multitargeted TKI of a number of intracellular signaling pathways involved in angiogenesis and tumor growth, such as VEGFR-2 and EGFR and REarranged during Transfection tyrosine kinase activity (95). It is currently FDA-approved for the treatment of unresectable, locally advanced or metastatic medullary thyroid cancer. There is a single-published phase II study investigating its efficacy as a single agent in the treatment of women with recurrent EOC (96). Unfortunately, it showed limited single-agent activity and was terminated in the first stage due to lack of response or disease stabilization beyond 6 months. Currently, there is a phase II trial underway investigating its efficacy in combination with liposomal doxorubicin for the treatment of recurrent EOC.

■ INHIBITORS OF THE PI3-KINASE/AKT/MTOR PATHWAY

The role of the PI3K/Akt/mTOR pathway in the development of cancer has been increasingly appreciated over the past decade as being important in carcinogenesis. Significant effort has been expended in developing targeted agents that block this pathway. Many types of amplified, overexpressed, and aberrant signaling elements throughout this pathway result in an increase in survival signaling. Hyperactive signaling through this pathway is also associated with resistance to chemotherapy and molecular targeting agents. All three elements of the pathway are either amplified or overexpressed in ovarian, endometrial, and cervical cancers, making this pathway an important target in gynecologic cancers.

This section focuses on the three primary players in this important pathway (recognizing that they all interact with and affect each other), the evidence that each is integral in different gynecologic malignancies, and the current developments in targeted agents. Given the complex interactions of Akt, PI3K, and mTOR, inhibition of any one of them will affect the others, either upstream or downstream; thus a discussion of any one of them is incomplete without including the others. Moreover, it has become increasingly evident that inhibiting one (or more than one) entry into this pathway is likely insufficient: the inhibitors will either need to be combined with cytotoxic chemotherapy, or combined with inhibitors of other pathways that may be turned on as a result of manipulation of the PI3K/Akt/mTOR pathway.

Akt

A serine/threonine protein kinase that plays a key role in multiple cellular processes including cell proliferation and apoptosis, Akt (also known as protein kinase B) is the primary mediator of the effects of PI3K (97). There are three members of the Akt family that have been identified: Akt1, Akt2, and Akt3. Akt1 inhibits apoptosis and is also able to induce protein synthesis. Akt2 is an important signaling molecule in the insulin signaling pathway. Akt3 may contribute to the aggressiveness of steroid hormone-insensitive cancers.

Akt has been found to be both activated and amplified in ovarian cancer. Yuan et al. demonstrated that 36% of ovarian cancers show elevated Akt2 activity (98). In vitro Akt2 kinase analysis in 91 ovarian cancer specimens revealed elevated levels of Akt2 activity (>3- fold) in 33 cases. The majority of tumors displaying activated Akt2 were of high grade and advanced stage. Akt3 is highly expressed in 21% of ovarian cancers (99).

In a study of Zorn et al. (100), immunostaining of an ovarian cancer tissue microarray revealed that 68% of ovarian carcinomas stained positive for phospho-Akt, suggesting that a higher percentage of ovarian cancers have activated Akt than previously thought. In addition, an association between phospho-Akt and phosphor-mTor staining was observed in 87% of ovarian tumors.

In cervical cancer, Liu et al. (101) demonstrated that the active metabolite of CPT-11, SN-38, inhibited cervical cell proliferation by down-regulating protein expression of phospho-Akt. Transfection of the full-length Akt cDNA resulted in the reduction of apoptosis caused by SN-28, and Akt kinase actively regulated the p53 pathway. The authors concluded that inhibition of the Akt pathway played an important role in the SN-38 cytotoxic effect in cervical cancer cells.

Nuclear p-Akt has been shown to be higher in endometrial cancer than in either normal endometrium or hyperplasia. In addition, the nuclear p-Akt of well-differentiated endometrial cancer is higher than that of moderately or poorly differentiated tumors. The nuclear expression of p-Akt correlates with that of the estrogen receptor alpha, and the level of nuclear p-Akt is significantly correlated with prognosis in grade 1 cancers (102). In another study, uterine sarcomas and grade 3 endometrioid endometrial cancers demonstrated higher levels of Akt compared with grade 1 endometrioid tumors. In cell lines, Akt cascade inhibitors decreased cell proliferation by apoptosis and cell cycle arrest (103). Most of the Akt inhibitors are still under development. None to date have been FDA approved.

KRX-0401 (Perifosine)

KRX-0401 (perifosine) is an oral agent that inhibits Akt activation. To date. more than 2,000 patients have been treated with KRX-0401 in clinical trials in the United States and Europe. The main side effects observed include nausea, vomiting, diarrhea, and fatigue. The drug has been studied in daily and weekly regimens.

Other Akt inhibitors under development include AT7867 (Astex Therapeutics, Cambridge, United Kingdom), GSK690693 (GlaxoSmithKline, San Diego, CA), MK-2206 (Merck, Whitehouse Station, NJ), and PHT-427 (PHusis Therapeutics, Houston, TX). Most of these drugs remain in preclinical development.

Phosphotidylinositol-3-kinase (PI3K)

PI3K is a lipid kinase that plays an important role in a wide variety of signaling pathways (97).

Amplification of PI3K has been shown to lead to paclitaxel resistance in ovarian cancer cells (104), a process that can be reversed by inhibitors of PI3K.

Cell biologist Lewis C. Cantley first discovered this kinase in 1985 (105), and it has been more than 10 years since the first compounds to block PI3K (LY294002 [Eli Lilly, Indianapolis, USA] and the natural product wortmannin) were reported (106). In recent years, several compounds have been developed that inhibit PI3K; many of these are combination inhibitors that also inhibit other members of the pathway.

PI3K is up-regulated in 30% to 45% of ovarian cancers (99,107). Interestingly, PI3K mutations vary by ovarian cancer histology. Only 2.3% of serous cancers have PI3K mutations compared with 20% of endometrioid and clear cell histologies suggesting that PI3K inhibitors may be particularly useful in the clear cell subtype (100). Unlike the mutation, however, PI3K gene amplification is common among all histologic subtypes. Overall, when considering mutation or gene amplification, abnormal PI3K expression is seen in 30% of ovarian cancers.

PI3K is a heterodimer composed of a catalytic subunit (p110a) encoded by PIK3CA and a regulatory subunit (p85a) encoded by PIK3R1. Two domains of p110a are frequently mutated in endometrial cancers (108). In addition, PIK3R1 is somatically mutated in 43% of endometrioid endometrial cancers and in 12% of nonendometrioid endometrial cancers (109). Several of these PIK3R1 mutations have been shown to promote increased phosphorylation of Akt, suggesting that targeted therapies directed against the PI3K pathway may be effective in endometrial cancer.

An in vivo study of cervical cancer cells revealed that PI3K inhibition enhanced radiosensitization. The combination of LY204002 and radiation resulted in significant and synergistic suppression of cervical cancer cells in a dose dependent manner via dephosphorylation of Akt. PI3K inhibition also suppressed tumor regrowth. These results suggest that this agent may be effective in future studies of cervical cancer and radiation (110).

The first generations of PI3K inhibitors are now entering midphase clinical trials. Many affect both the PI3K family of enzymes and mTOR (see below). Several large pharmaceutical companies have already developed dual mTOR/PI3K inhibitors that are in clinical trials.

SF1126

Semafore Pharmaceuticals (Westfield, IN) was one of the first companies to develop a dual mTOR/PI3K inhibitor. Semafore scientists developed a prodrug of LY294002, called SF1126, that delivers the active molecule to solid tumors. Phase I studies of the prodrug, which can be administered at higher concentrations than LY294002 without the same toxicity problems, have been completed.

PX-886

PX-886 is most selective for the α- and β-isoforms of PI3K. The compound is being tested in combination with other therapies in two phase I/II trials, including a study of its effectiveness with Erbitux (ImClone Inc., East Bridgewater, NJ) in the treatment of colon cancer.

GDC 0941

GDC 0941 is a PI3K inhibitor currently in phase I trials in solid tumors and non-Hodgkins lymphoma. Phase Ib trials for metastatic breast cancer and metastatic non–small cell lung cancer are ongoing evaluating GDC 0941 in combination with bevacizumab, trastuzumab, and erlotinib. A phase II clinical trial evaluating both GDC 0941 and GDC 0980 in combination with hormones for second-line ER-positive metastatic breast cancer is also ongoing. GDC 0941 is being studied in combination with paclitaxel (and carboplatin) and bevacizumab for breast cancer. Other PI3 kinase inhibitors are currently under development.

mTOR (Protein Mammalian Target of Rapamycin)

mTOR is a conserved serine-threonine kinase that regulates cell growth and metabolism. Aberrant high activity of mTOR is associated with human gynecologic cancers. Downstream from Akt and PI3K, mTOR plays a critical role in transducing proliferative signals mediated through the PI3K pathway. It also plays a fundamental role in other critical cellular functions that affect cell growth and proliferation. Activation of the mTOR pathway occurs frequently in gynecologic cancers, particularly in ovarian and endometrial cancers. Aberrant phosphorylation of PTEN has been detected in more than 70% of endometrial cancers (111).

Inhibition of mTOR abolishes the proliferative and nutrient utilization signals, resulting in cell cycle arrest and tumor growth inhibition. The prototypic mTOR inhibitor is rapamycin. However, rapamycin has a poor pharmacologic profile, including poor water solubility. Thus, other mTOR inhibitors have been developed for clinical use, including CCI-779 (temsirolimus), RAD001 (everolimus), and AP23573 (ARIAD, deforolimus).

IHC analysis revealed that mTOR activity was much higher in cervical cancers than in normal cervical tissue. In invasive cervical squamous carcinomas, the expression of mTOR gradually increased with increasing degree of malignancy. These results suggest that overactivation of the mTOR gene plays an important role in the pathogenesis of human cervical carcinoma. Rapamycin also inhibited the activation of the mTOR pathway in all four cervical cancer cell lines tested (112).

Dysregulation of the mTOR pathway has been demonstrated in ovarian cancer in general and clear cell carcinomas of the ovary specifically (113–115). Efforts to inhibit mTOR signaling to arrest progress of cells through the cell cycle can also lead to inhibition of angiogenesis. In an evaluation of tissue microarrays of 98 primary ovarian cancers (52 clear cell carcinomas and 46 serous adenocarcinomas), the expression of phospho-mTOR was assessed (114). Then, the growth-inhibitory effect of mTOR inhibition by RAD001 was examined using human clear cell carcinoma cell lines. IHC analysis revealed that mTOR was more frequently activated in clear cell carcinomas than in serous adenocarcinomas (86.6% vs. 50%). Treatment with RAD001 markedly inhibited the growth of clear cell carcinoma cell lines both in vitro and in vivo. Increased expression of phospho-mTOR was observed in cisplatin-resistant clear cell carcinoma cell lines, compared with respective parental cells. This increased expression of phospho-mTOR in cisplatin-resistant cells was associated with increased activation of Akt (114). This study found that mTOR is frequently activated in clear cell carcinoma and could be a promising therapeutic target in the management of these patients.

Endometrial Cancer and PTEN

Loss of PTEN function is an early event in type I endometrial cancer. When PTEN is deleted, mutated or inactivated, activation of Akt and mTOR can occur and tumorigenesis can be initiated. Inactivation of the PTEN tumor-suppressor gene is the most common genetic defect in endometrial cancers (111).

PTEN is a tumor suppressor gene encoding a lipid phosphatase which acts to maintain G1 arrest and enable apoptosis through an Akt-dependent mechanism (116,117). PTEN acts in opposition to PIK3CA to control levels of phosphorylated Akt. PIK3CA mutation, seen in 36% of endometrial carcinomas is most frequent in tumors which also have a PTEN mutation (118). The lack of functional PTEN leads to activation of downstream components of the mTOR pathway, including Akt. mTOR inhibition is therefore a rational targeted therapy for endometrial cancer.

The tumor suppressor p53 activates the transcription of PTEN and therefore functions as a negative regulator of the entire PI3K signaling pathway. When both PTEN and p53 pathways are inactivated by mutations, malignancy is promoted synergistically. Ras and its downstream effectors can activate components of the PI3K pathway through numerous mechanisms.

Temsirolimus, Deforolimus, and Everolimus

Three mTOR inhibitors (temsirolimus [CCI-779], deforolimus [AP23573, MK-8669], and everolimus [rad001]) are in clinical trials focusing on endometrial cancer. Preliminary results of a phase II trial of temsirolimus in recurrent or metastatic endometrial cancer (chemotherapy naïve, with up to one prior line of hormonal therapy) demonstrated encouraging results with 5 of 19 evaluable patients (26%) achieving a PR (119). Three PR patients had papillary serous tumors.

A phase II trial of everolimus at MD Anderson Cancer Center in patients with one or two prior chemotherapy regimens reported a clinical benefit rate (stable disease > 8 weeks) of 44% (11 of 25 evaluable patients) (120,121). Entry was limited to women with endometrioid histology. A phase II trial of deforolimus in recurrent or metastatic endometrial cancer and carcinosarcoma of the uterus (with up to two prior cytotoxic regimens) revealed a response rate of 9% (4 of 45 evaluable patients) (122). Responses were seen in endometrioid (2), papillary serous (1), and clear cell (1) histologies. A phase I trial of paclitaxel, carboplatin, and temsirolimus has been completed (NCI study NCT00408655).

The GOG has completed one study of temsirolimus in recurrent or persistent endometrial cancer: GOG 229G was a Phase II Evaluation of Combination Bevacizumab (NCI-Supplied Agent: NSC #704865, IND #7921) and Temsirolimus (CCI-779, NCI-Supplied Agent: NSC #683864, IND #61010) in the treatment of recurrent or persistent endometrial carcinoma.

A randomized phase II trial of temsirolimus or the combination of hormonal therapy plus temsirolimus in women with advanced, persistent, or recurrent endometrial carcinoma, GOG 248 recently completed accrual. A three-arm randomized phase II study, GOG86P compared paclitaxel/carboplatin/bevacizumab, paclitaxel/carboplatin/temsirilomus, and ixabepilone/carboplatin/bevacizumab as initial therapy in measurable disease stage III or IVA, stage IVB, or recurrent endometrial cancer.

There is evidence that mTOR inhibitors have activity in ovarian cancer. The results of GOG 170I were presented at the Society of Gynecologic Oncologists (SGO) in 2010. Sixty women with up to three prior chemotherapy regimens were enrolled on this phase II study. Of the 54 evaluable patients, 24% had a PFS ≥6 months, 9% achieved a PR, and 41% had stable disease, for a combined response rate of 74%. The median PFS and OS were 3.2 and 11.6 months, respectively. Toxicities included metabolic toxicities, nausea, pain, anemia, and infection.

Temsirolimus has been tested as a single agent in patients with recurrent ovarian carcinoma and in a phase I trial in combination with carboplatin and paclitaxel (123,124). A 3+3 dose-escalation phase I study has been conducted in patients with advanced solid malignancies suitable for carboplatin and paclitaxel chemotherapy who had not received more than two prior chemotherapy regimens (124). To date, 31 eligible patients with a median age of 59 years have been treated and 27 are evaluable for toxicity. Patients were entered in six dose levels, with the first two levels receiving temsirolimus on days 8 and 15 and the next 4 levels switching to days 1 and 8. This dose-escalation phase I study found that administration of temsirolimus on days 8 and 15 was not feasible due to myelosuppression on day 15. The combination of carboplatin and paclitaxel on day 1 with temsirolimus on days 1 and 8 was well tolerated, and patients have received a median of five cycles of therapy. At dose level 6 (temsirolimus 25 mg days 1 and 8, paclitaxel 175 mg/m^2 day 1, carboplatin AUC 6 day 1) dose limiting toxicity (DLT) was seen in one of six patients treated to date (grade 4 thrombocytopenia) and a second patient had a possible DLT (grade 3 fatigue in presence of baseline fatigue) (124). Of the 26 patients with follow-up data, there have been 10 (38.5%) partial responders with a median duration of 7.1 months, and 12 (46%) with stable disease. The results indicated that this combination was well tolerated and requires additional assessment in a phase II setting.

A phase II evaluation of temsirolimus in combination with carboplatin and paclitaxel followed by temsirolimus consolidation as first-line therapy in the treatment of clear cell carcinoma of the ovary, GOG 268 is currently accruing patients.

mTOR inhibitors are being studied in all gynecologic cancers. There are many other open investigations in gynecologic cancers.

■ OTHER AGENTS

Aurora Kinase Inhibitors

The aurora kinase family is a collection of highly related serine-threonine kinases that are key regulators of mitosis. There are three members: A, B, and C. Deregulation of aurora kinases has been linked to tumorigenesis and aurora kinase A is most often associated with malignancy (125).

Aurora kinase A and aurora kinase B are overexpressed in some gynecologic cancers, and their overexpression is associated with poor prognosis (126). In particular, aurora kinase A has been significantly associated with tumor grade, tumor stage, and survival (127). In addition, in a small study from MD Anderson Cancer Center, it was demonstrated that aurora kinase A regulates genomic instability and tumorigenesis through cell cycle dysregulation and BRCA2 suppression in ovarian cancer cell lines (128).

Most of the current data on aurora kinases is preclinical. The company Millennium (Takeda Pharmaceutical Company, Osaka, Japan) is investigating the aurora kinase MLN8237 in patients with ovarian cancer in a phase I/II design.

PARP Inhibitors

Poly (ADP-ribose) polymerase (PARP) is another target for developing agents for the treatment of ovarian cancer. PARP plays a critical role in base excision repair of single-strand DNA breaks. By inhibiting

PARP, single-strand DNA breaks accumulate, which can lead to double-strand DNA breaks. Double strand DNA breaks are typically repaired by the homologous recombination repair pathway. The tumor suppressor genes BRCA1 and BRCA2 are vital components of that pathway (129). About 10% of women with ovarian cancer carry a BRCA1 or a BRCA2 mutation and it is estimated that up to 50% and 60% of women with high-grade EOC may have functional loss of proteins involved in the homologous recombination repair pathway of DNA repair and thus have tumors that behave in a manner similar to BRCA 1/2 mutant cancers (130–132). Therefore, ovarian cancer cells are more dependent on single-strand DNA repair processes. PARP is crucial for single-strand DNA repair and could prevent cells with abnormal BRCA function (like ovarian cancer cells) from repairing chemotherapy induced DNA damage and thus may increase the cytotoxicity of chemotherapeutic agents (133). There are currently several PARP inhibitors currently in clinical trial for the treatment of ovarian cancer including, olaparib (AZD2281) veliparib (ABT-888), MK-4827, and AG-014699.

A phase II trial investigated the use of olaparib for patients with BRCA1 or BRCA2 mutations and recurrent ovarian cancer (134). Two sequential cohorts were enrolled. The first cohort (n = 33) received 400 mg twice daily and the second cohort (n = 24) received 100 mg twice daily. The objective response rate was 11 of 33 (33%) in the cohort receiving 400 mg twice daily and 3 of 24 (13%) in patients receiving 100 mg twice daily. The most common side effects were nausea and fatigue. Overall, olaparib was well tolerated and resulted in a favorable response rate in this highly pretreated population.

The use of olaparib has also been investigated in unselected patient populations. A phase II study of women with advanced ovarian cancer demonstrated evidence of single-agent activity among women with high-grade serous ovarian cancer unselected for the presence of a germline BRCA mutation (135). There are currently ongoing clinical trials examining the use of olaparib and veliparib in the treatment of newly diagnosed and recurrent ovarian cancer in combination with other agents including the antiangiogenic agent cediranib (136) and carboplatin (137).

Hedgehog Inhibitors

Hedgehog (HH) proteins consist of a small family of intercellular signaling molecules. In humans, there are three HH proteins: sonic HH (Shh), Indian HH (Ihh), and desert HH (Dhh). The transmembrane protein receptor Patched functions as a tumor suppressor that inhibits Smoothened (Smo) from activating downstream signaling. Activation of the pathway is initiated through binding of any of the three HH proteins to Patched. Aberrant activation of the HH signaling pathway has been reported in human cancers such as basal cell carcinoma, prostate cancer, and ovarian cancer (138,139).

Several groups have demonstrated that HH signaling is active in human ovarian cancer cell lines. One group used human ovarian cancer cell lines to demonstrate that HH signaling is active in human ovarian cancer and responsible for both clonal growth and proliferation (139). Liao et al., using both ovarian tumor samples and cell lines, demonstrated that overexpression of Patched in ovarian cancers correlated with poor survival. Elevated Shh messenger RNA was observed more frequently in ovarian cancers compared with normal ovarian tissue (138). Rueda et al. (140) reported that 50% of ovarian cancer samples expressed Shh in the tumor epithelium. These investigators then used human serous ovarian cancer xenograft tissue to create a mouse model that they treated with an HH inhibitor, with and without the addition of chemotherapy. In both the active treatment and the maintenance phase of the experiment, the HH inhibitor was shown to inhibit growth of the tumor.

GDC-449 is an HH inhibitor that was studied in ovarian cancer in a phase II study of GDC-449 as maintenance therapy in patients with ovarian cancer in a second or third complete remission. Results are not yet available.

■ IMMUNOTHERAPY

The emerging role of immunotherapy in the treatment of ovarian cancer and other gynecologic malignancies has been well-summarized in recent reviews (141–144). Interested readers are referred to these review articles for in depth summaries of the topic. Examples of the various approaches to immunotherapy and details about current immunotherapy techniques being used in clinical trials are discussed here. There are several basic approaches to use the immunotherapy in cancer treatment, including the use of monoclonal antibodies and antibody-based immunotherapy, adoptive immunotherapy, and tumor vaccine therapy.

Monoclonal Antibody Therapy

Monoclonal antibodies can induce antitumor effects by interacting with tumor cell surface signaling proteins or other serum proteins such as VEGF. After binding to their targets, antibodies exercise their function by means of several different mechanisms including complement activation, directly inducing antiproliferative effects and activation of cell-mediated cytotoxicity (145). Several of the agents previously mentioned in this review article are monoclonal antibodies, such as bevacizumab, trastuzumab, and cetuximab.

Another example of a monoclonal antibody currently in clinical trials for the treatment of gynecologic malignancies is farletuzumab. Farletuzumab is a humanized IGg1 monoclonal antibody that targets the human folate receptor alpha (146). This receptor is overexpressed in most EOCs and its overexpression is associated with stage and grade of disease (147). A phase I study of women with platinum-refractory or -resistant EOC assessing the use of farletuzumab as single-agent therapy demonstrated that the drug is safe and well tolerated in this heavily pretreated population (148). Final data from a multicenter phase II trial evaluating the use of farletuzumab in conjunction with carboplatin and taxane in women with platinum-sensitive EOC in first relapse were recently presented (149). Farletuzumab was well tolerated and 89% of evaluable subjects had normalization of their CA-125 levels. There are phase II and III trials currently recruiting patients evaluating the use of farletuzumab in combination with cytotoxic chemotherapy.

Adoptive Immunotherapy

Adoptive immunotherapy is a treatment approach consisting of the ex vivo expansion of antitumor immune cells followed by the administration of these effector cells to a tumor-bearing host (150). Early approaches using adoptive immunity for the treatment of ovarian cancer used peripheral blood monocytes exposed to IL-2 ex vivo, which led to the generation of lymphokine-activated killer (LAK) cells that were cytotoxic for a variety of tumor cells (151). Experimental treatments using this technique did yield some responses, but a great deal of toxicity was seen (151–153). More recently, the use of ex vivo expanded tumor infiltrating lymphocytes (TILs) has produced promising clinical results (143).

Tumor Vaccine Therapy

In ovarian cancer and a number of other tumor types, vaccines have been the main approach to immunotherapy. Current efforts to improve vaccines are directed at optimizing the choice of antigens, improving delivery systems and developing combination approaches (143).

For example, GOG 255 is a randomized phase III trial currently enrolling patients evaluating vaccine therapy and OPT-821, a vaccine adjuvant, to see how well this combination works compared with OPT-821 alone in women with EOC, FTC, or PPC in their second or third complete clinical remission. In one arm, patients receive both polyvalent antigen-KLH conjugate vaccine in combination with OPT-821 and in the second arm patients receive only OPT-821.

■ SUMMARY

There has been a recent rapid increase in the number of targeted therapies under development for gynecologic malignancies. Many of the agents tested have not demonstrated robust clinical responses or improvements in patient survival. However, trials involving targeted agents must be interpreted carefully as these agents may be important in future trials that have a more rational design. Moreover, the traditional measures of response used for chemotherapy (such as RECIST, for example) may not apply to the biologics, making an accurate measure of response with these drugs challenging. Future directions include testing targeted therapies in combination with other agents and in more highly selected patient populations.

■ REFERENCES

1. Hanahan D, Weinberg RA. The hallmarks of cancer. *Cell*. 2000;100(1):57–70.

2. Burger RA. Role of vascular endothelial growth factor inhibitors in the treatment of gynecologic malignancies. *J Gynecol Oncol*. 2010;21(1):3–11.

3. Frederick PJ, Straughn JM, Jr., Alvarez RD, et al. Preclinical studies and clinical utilization of monoclonal antibodies in epithelial ovarian cancer. *Gynecol Oncol*. 2009;113(3):384–390.

4. Frumovitz M, Sood AK. Vascular endothelial growth factor (VEGF) pathway as a therapeutic target in gynecologic malignancies. *Gynecol Oncol*. 2007;104(3):768–778.

5. Han ES, Lin P, Wakabayashi M. Current status on biologic therapies in the treatment of epithelial ovarian cancer. *Curr Treat Options Oncol*. 2009;10(1–2):54–66.

6. Folkman J. What is the evidence that tumors are angiogenesis dependent? *J Natl Cancer Inst*. 1990;82(1):4–6.

7. Gordon MS, Margolin K, Talpaz M, et al. Phase I safety and pharmacokinetic study of recombinant human anti-vascular endothelial growth factor in patients with advanced cancer. *J Clin Oncol*. 2001;19(3):843–850.

8. Hurwitz H, Fehrenbacher L, Novotny W, et al. Bevacizumab plus irinotecan, fluorouracil, and leucovorin for metastatic colorectal cancer. *N Engl J Med*. 2004;350(23):2335–2342.

9. Giantonio BJ, Catalano PJ, Meropol NJ, et al. Bevacizumab in combination with oxaliplatin, fluorouracil, and leucovorin (FOLFOX4) for previously treated metastatic colorectal cancer: Results from the Eastern Cooperative Oncology Group Study E3200. *J Clin Oncol*. 2007;25(12):1539–1544.

10. Tebbutt NC, Wilson K, Gebski VJ, et al. Capecitabine, bevacizumab, and mitomycin in first-line treatment of metastatic colorectal cancer: results of the Australasian Gastrointestinal Trials Group Randomized Phase III MAX Study. *J Clin Oncol*. 2010;28(19):3191–3198.

11. Miller K, Wang M, Gralow J, et al. Paclitaxel plus bevacizumab versus paclitaxel alone for metastatic breast cancer. *N Engl J Med*. 2007;357(26):2666–2676.

12. Miles DW, Chan A, Dirix LY, et al. Phase III study of bevacizumab plus docetaxel compared with placebo plus docetaxel for the first-line treatment of human epidermal growth factor receptor 2-negative metastatic breast cancer. *J Clin Oncol*. 2010;28(20):3239–3247.

13. Robert NJ, Dieras V, Glaspy J, et al. RIBBON-1: Randomized, double-blind, placebo-controlled, phase III trial of chemotherapy with or without bevacizumab for first-line treatment of human epidermal growth factor receptor 2-negative, locally recurrent or metastatic breast cancer. *J Clin Oncol*. 2011;29(10):1252–1260.

14. Sandler A, Gray R, Perry MC, et al. Paclitaxel-carboplatin alone or with bevacizumab for non-small-cell lung cancer. *N Engl J Med*. 2006;355(24):2542–2550.

15. Reck M, von Pawel J, Zatloukal P, et al. Phase III trial of cisplatin plus gemcitabine with either placebo or bevacizumab as first-line therapy for nonsquamous non-small-cell lung cancer: AVAil. *J Clin Oncol*. 2009;27(8):1227–1234.

16. Reck M, von Pawel J, Zatloukal P, et al. Overall survival with cisplatin-gemcitabine and bevacizumab or placebo as first-line therapy for nonsquamous non-small-cell lung cancer: Results from a randomised phase III trial (AVAiL). *Ann Oncol*. 2010;21(9):1804–1809.

17. *FDA Approval for Bevacizumab*. http://www.cancer.gov/cancertopics/druginfo/fda-bevacizumab. Updated 2010. Accessed 05/30, 2011.

18. Burger RA, Sill MW, Monk BJ, et al. Phase II trial of bevacizumab in persistent or recurrent epithelial ovarian cancer or primary peritoneal cancer: A Gynecologic Oncology Group Study. *J Clin Oncol.* 2007;25(33):5165–5171.

19. Cannistra SA, Matulonis UA, Penson RT, et al. Phase II study of bevacizumab in patients with platinum-resistant ovarian cancer or peritoneal serous cancer. *J Clin Oncol.* 2007;25(33):5180–5186.

20. Burger RA, Brady MF, Bookman MA, et al. Phase III trial of bevacizumab (BEV) in the primary treatment of advanced epithelial ovarian cancer (EOC), primary peritoneal cancer (PPC), or fallopian tube cancer (FTC): A Gynecologic Oncology Group study. *J Clin Oncol.* 2010;28(18):LBA1.

21. ICON 7: *Bevacizumab in ovarian cancer.* http://www.icon7trial.org/. Accessed 05/30, 2011.

22. Aghajanian C, Finkler NJ, Rutherford T, et al. OCEANS: A randomized, double-blinded, placebo-controlled phase III trial of chemotherapy with or without bevacizumab (BEV) in patients with platinum-sensitive recurrent epithelial ovarian (EOC), primary peritoneal (PPC), or fallopian tube cancer (FTC). *ASCO Meeting Abstracts.* 2011;29(18, suppl):LBA5007.

23. Han ES, Monk BJ. What is the risk of bowel perforation associated with bevacizumab therapy in ovarian cancer? *Gynecol Oncol.* 2007;105(1):3–6.

24. Randall LM, Monk BJ. Bevacizumab toxicities and their management in ovarian cancer. *Gynecol Oncol.* 2010;117(3):497–504.

25. Gurevich F, Perazella MA. Renal effects of anti-angiogenesis therapy: update for the internist. *Am J Med.* 2009;122(4):322–328.

26. Holash J, Davis S, Papadopoulos N, et al. VEGF-Trap: A VEGF blocker with potent antitumor effects. *Proc Natl Acad Sci U S A.* 2002;99(17):11393–11398.

27. Byrne AT, Ross L, Holash J, et al. Vascular endothelial growth factor-trap decreases tumor burden, inhibits ascites, and causes dramatic vascular remodeling in an ovarian cancer model. *Clin Cancer Res.* 2003;9(15):5721–5728.

28. Leighl NB, Raez LE, Besse B, et al. A multicenter, phase 2 study of vascular endothelial growth factor trap (Aflibercept) in platinum- and erlotinib-resistant adenocarcinoma of the lung. *J Thorac Oncol.* 2010;5(7):1054–1059.

29. Twardowski P, Stadler WM, Frankel P, et al. Phase II study of Aflibercept (VEGF-Trap) in patients with recurrent or metastatic urothelial cancer, a California Cancer Consortium Trial. *Urology.* 2010;76(4):923–926.

30. Tew WP, Colombo N, Ray-Coquard I, et al. VEGF-Trap for patients (pts) with recurrent platinum-resistant epithelial ovarian cancer (EOC): Preliminary results of a randomized, multicenter phase II study (abstr. 5508). *J Clin Oncol.* 2007;25(18S):276s.

31. Coleman RL, Duska LR, Ramirez PT, et al. Phase II multi-institutional study of docetaxel plus aflibercept (AVE0005, NSC# 724770) in patients with recurrent ovarian, primary peritoneal, and fallopian tube cancer. *ASCO Meeting Abstracts.* 2011;29(15, suppl):5017.

32. Izzedine H, Buhaescu I, Rixe O, Deray G. Sunitinib malate. *Cancer Chemother Pharmacol.* 2007;60(3):357–364.

33. Hensley ML, Sill MW, Scribner DR, Jr., et al. Sunitinib malate in the treatment of recurrent or persistent uterine leiomyosarcoma: A Gynecologic Oncology Group phase II study. *Gynecol Oncol.* 2009;115(3):460–465.

34. Welch S, Hirte H, Schilder RJ, et al. Phase II study of sorafenib (BAY 43–9006) in combination with gemcitabine in recurrent epithelial ovarian cancer: A PMH phase II consortium trial. *ASCO Meeting Abstracts.* 2006;24(18, suppl):5084.

35. Welch S, Mackay HJ, Hirte H, et al. A phase II study of sunitinib in recurrent or metastatic endometrial carcinoma: A trial of the PMH Phase II Consortium. *ASCO Meeting Abstracts.* 2009;27(15S):5576.

36. Correa R, Mackay H, Hirte HW, et al. A phase II study of sunitinib in recurrent or metastatic endometrial carcinoma: A trial of the Princess Margaret Hospital, The University of Chicago, and California Cancer Phase II Consortia. *ASCO Meeting Abstracts.* 2010;28(15, suppl):5038.

37. Biagi JJ, Oza AM, Grimshaw R, et al. A phase II study of sunitinib (SU11248) in patients (pts) with recurrent epithelial ovarian, fallopian tube or primary peritoneal carcinoma—NCIC CTG IND 185. *ASCO Meeting Abstracts.* 2008;26(15, suppl):5522.

38. Sonpavde G, Hutson TE. Pazopanib: A novel multitargeted tyrosine kinase inhibitor. *Curr Oncol Rep.* 2007;9(2):115–119.

39. Friedlander M, Hancock KC, Rischin D, et al. A Phase II, open-label study evaluating pazopanib in patients with recurrent ovarian cancer. *Gynecol Oncol.* 2010;119(1):32–37.

40. Monk BJ, Mas Lopez L, Zarba JJ, et al. Phase II, open-label study of pazopanib or lapatinib monotherapy compared with pazopanib plus lapatinib combination therapy in patients with advanced and recurrent cervical cancer. *J Clin Oncol.* 2010;28(22):3562–3569.

41. Dempke WC, Zippel R. Brivanib, a novel dual VEGF-R2/bFGF-R inhibitor. *Anticancer Res.* 2010;30(11):4477–4483.

42. Garrett CR, Siu LL, El-Khoueiry A, et al. Phase I dose-escalation study to determine the safety, pharmacokinetics and pharmacodynamics of brivanib alaninate in combination with full-dose cetuximab in patients with advanced gastrointestinal malignancies who have failed prior therapy. *Br J Cancer.* 2011;105(1):44–52.

43. Jonker DJ, Rosen LS, Sawyer MB, et al. A phase I study to determine the safety, pharmacokinetics and pharmacodynamics of a dual VEGFR and FGFR inhibitor, brivanib, in patients with advanced or metastatic solid tumors. *Ann Oncol.* 2011;22(6):1413–1419.

44. Brave SR, Ratcliffe K, Wilson Z, et al. Assessing the Activity of Cediranib, a VEGFR-2/3 Tyrosine Kinase Inhibitor, against VEGFR-1 and Members of the Structurally Related PDGFR Family. *Mol Cancer Ther.* 2011;10(5):861–873.

45. Hess-Stumpp H, Haberey M, Thierauch KH. PTK 787/ZK 222584, a tyrosine kinase inhibitor of all known VEGF receptors, represses tumor growth with high efficacy. *Chembiochem.* 2005;6(3):550–557.

46. Hilberg F, Roth GJ, Krssak M, et al. BIBF 1120: triple angiokinase inhibitor with sustained receptor blockade and good antitumor efficacy. *Cancer Res.* 2008;68(12): 4774–4782.

47. Matulonis UA, Berlin S, Ivy P, et al. Cediranib, an oral inhibitor of vascular endothelial growth factor receptor kinases, is an active drug in recurrent epithelial ovarian, fallopian tube, and peritoneal cancer. *J Clin Oncol.* 2009;27(33):5601–5606.

48. Juretzka MM, Aghajanian C, Hensley ML, et al. Phase I trial of PTK787/ZK222584 (PTK/ZK) in combination with carboplatin (C) and paclitaxel (T) in platinum-sensitive recurrent epithelial ovarian (EOC), fallopian tube (FT), or primary peritoneal (PPC) cancers. *ASCO Meeting Abstracts.* 2007;25(18, suppl):5564.

49. Schroder W, Campone M, Abadie S, et al. A phase IB, open label, safety and pharmacokinetic (PK) study of escalating doses of PTK787/ZK 222584 (PTK/ZK) in combination with paclitaxel and carboplatin in patients (Pts) with stage IC to IV epithelial ovarian cancer (EOC). *ASCO Meeting Abstracts.* 2006;24(18, suppl):5075.

50. du Bois A, Huober J, Stopfer P, et al. A phase I open-label dose-escalation study of oral BIBF 1120 combined with standard paclitaxel and carboplatin in patients with advanced gynecological malignancies. *Ann Oncol.* 2010;21(2):370–375.

51. Ledermann JA, Rustin GJ, Hackshaw A, et al. A randomized phase II placebo-controlled trial using maintenance therapy to evaluate the vascular targeting agent BIBF 1120 following treatment of relapsed ovarian cancer (OC). *ASCO Meeting Abstracts.* 2009;27(15S):5501.

52. de Bono JS, Rowinsky EK. The ErbB receptor family: A therapeutic target for cancer. *Trends Mol Med.* 2002; 8(4 Suppl):S19–S26.

53. Ciardiello F, Tortora G. A novel approach in the treatment of cancer: targeting the epidermal growth factor receptor. *Clin Cancer Res.* 2001;7(10):2958–2970.

54. Palayekar MJ, Herzog TJ. The emerging role of epidermal growth factor receptor inhibitors in ovarian cancer. *Int J Gynecol Cancer.* 2008;18(5):879–890.

55. Arteaga CL. The epidermal growth factor receptor: From mutant oncogene in nonhuman cancers to therapeutic target in human neoplasia. *J Clin Oncol.* 2001; 19(18 Suppl):32S–40S.

56. Baselga J. The EGFR as a target for anticancer therapy—focus on cetuximab. *Eur J Cancer.* 2001;37 Suppl 4:S16–22.

57. Schilder RJ, Pathak HB, Lokshin AE, et al. Phase II trial of single agent cetuximab in patients with persistent or recurrent epithelial ovarian or primary peritoneal carcinoma with the potential for dose escalation to rash. *Gynecol Oncol.* 2009;113(1):21–27.

58. Konner J, Schilder RJ, DeRosa FA, et al. A phase II study of cetuximab/paclitaxel/carboplatin for the initial treatment of advanced-stage ovarian, primary peritoneal, or fallopian tube cancer. *Gynecol Oncol.* 2008;110(2): 140–145.

59. Secord AA, Blessing JA, Armstrong DK, et al. Phase II trial of cetuximab and carboplatin in relapsed platinum-sensitive ovarian cancer and evaluation of epidermal growth factor receptor expression: A Gynecologic Oncology Group study. *Gynecol Oncol.* 2008;108(3):493–499.

60. Farley J, Sill MW, Birrer M, et al. Phase II study of cisplatin plus cetuximab in advanced, recurrent, and previously treated cancers of the cervix and evaluation of epidermal growth factor receptor immunohistochemical expression: A Gynecologic Oncology Group study. *Gynecol Oncol.* 2011;121(2):303–308.

61. Moore KN, Sill M, Miller DS, et al. A phase I trial of concurrent cetuximab (CET), cisplatin (CDDP), and radiation therapy (RT) women with locally advanced cervical cancer (CXCA): A GOG study. *ASCO Meeting Abstracts.* 2011;29(15, suppl):5032.

62. Bookman MA, Darcy KM, Clarke-Pearson D, Boothby RA, Horowitz IR. Evaluation of monoclonal humanized anti-HER2 antibody, trastuzumab, in patients with recurrent or refractory ovarian or primary peritoneal carcinoma with overexpression of HER2: A phase II trial of the Gynecologic Oncology Group. *J Clin Oncol.* 2003;21(2):283–290.

63. Fleming GF, Sill MW, Darcy KM, et al. Phase II trial of trastuzumab in women with advanced or recurrent, HER2-positive endometrial carcinoma: A Gynecologic Oncology Group study. *Gynecol Oncol.* 2010;116(1):15–20.

64. Rudin CM, Liu W, Desai A, et al. Pharmacogenomic and pharmacokinetic determinants of erlotinib toxicity. *J Clin Oncol.* 2008;26(7):1119–1127.

65. Gordon AN, Finkler N, Edwards RP, et al. Efficacy and safety of erlotinib HCl, an epidermal growth factor receptor (HER1/EGFR) tyrosine kinase inhibitor, in patients with advanced ovarian carcinoma: Results from a phase II multicenter study. *Int J Gynecol Cancer.* 2005;15(5):785–792.

66. Nimeiri HS, Oza AM, Morgan RJ, et al. Efficacy and safety of bevacizumab plus erlotinib for patients with recurrent ovarian, primary peritoneal, and fallopian tube cancer: A trial of the Chicago, PMH, and California Phase II Consortia. *Gynecol Oncol.* 2008;110(1):49–55.

67. Vasey PA, Gore M, Wilson R, et al. A phase Ib trial of docetaxel, carboplatin and erlotinib in ovarian, fallopian tube and primary peritoneal cancers. *Br J Cancer.* 2008;98(11):1774–1780.

68. Hirte H, Oza A, Swenerton K, et al. A phase II study of erlotinib (OSI-774) given in combination with carboplatin in patients with recurrent epithelial ovarian cancer (NCIC CTG IND.149). *Gynecol Oncol.* 2010;118(3):308–312.

69. Chambers SK, Clouser MC, Baker AF, et al. Overexpression of tumor vascular endothelial growth factor A may portend an increased likelihood of progression in a phase II trial of bevacizumab and erlotinib in resistant ovarian cancer. *Clin Cancer Res.* 2010;16(21):5320–5328.

70. Blank SV, Christos P, Curtin JP, et al. Erlotinib added to carboplatin and paclitaxel as first-line treatment of ovarian cancer: A phase II study based on surgical reassessment. *Gynecol Oncol.* 2010;119(3):451–456.

71. Schilder RJ, Sill MW, Lee YC, Mannel R. A phase II trial of erlotinib in recurrent squamous cell carcinoma of the cervix: A Gynecologic Oncology Group Study. *Int J Gynecol Cancer.* 2009;19(5):929–933.

72. Schilder RJ, Sill MW, Chen X, et al. Phase II study of gefitinib in patients with relapsed or persistent ovarian or primary peritoneal carcinoma and evaluation of epidermal growth factor receptor mutations and immunohistochemical expression: A Gynecologic Oncology Group Study. *Clin Cancer Res.* 2005;11(15):5539–5548.

73. Pautier P, Joly F, Kerbrat P, et al. Phase II study of gefitinib in combination with paclitaxel (P) and carboplatin (C) as second-line therapy for ovarian, tubal or peritoneal adenocarcinoma (1839IL/0074). *Gynecol Oncol.* 2010;116(2):157–162.

74. Goncalves A, Fabbro M, Lhomme C, et al. A phase II trial to evaluate gefitinib as second- or third-line treatment in patients with recurring locoregionally advanced or metastatic cervical cancer. *Gynecol Oncol.* 2008;108(1):42–46.

75. Leslie KK, Sill MW, Darcy KM, et al. Efficacy and safety of gefitinib and potential prognostic value of soluble EGFR, EGFR mutations, and tumor markers in a Gynecologic Oncology Group phase II trial of persistent or recurrent endometrial cancer. *ASCO Meeting Abstracts.* 2009;27(15S):e16542.

76. Medina PJ, Goodin S. Lapatinib: A dual inhibitor of human epidermal growth factor receptor tyrosine kinases. *Clin Ther.* 2008;30(8):1426–1447.

77. Kimball KJ, Numnum TM, Kirby TO, et al. A phase I study of lapatinib in combination with carboplatin in women with platinum sensitive recurrent ovarian carcinoma. *Gynecol Oncol.* 2008;111(1):95–101.

78. Rivkin SE, Muller C, Iriarte D, Arthur J, Canoy A, Reid H. Phase I/II lapatinib plus carboplatin and paclitaxel in stage III or IV relapsed ovarian cancer patients. *ASCO Meeting Abstracts.* 2008;26(15, suppl):5556.

79. Weroha SJ, Oberg AL, Ziegler KL, et al. Phase II trial of lapatinib and topotecan (LapTop) in patients with platinum-refractory/resistant ovarian and primary peritoneal carcinoma. *Gynecol Oncol.* 2011;122(1):116–120.

80. Dushkin H, Schilder RJ. Imatinib mesylate and its potential implications for gynecologic cancers. *Curr Treat Options Oncol.* 2005;6(2):115–120.

81. Schmandt RE, Broaddus R, Lu KH, et al. Expression of c-ABL, c-KIT, and platelet-derived growth factor receptor-beta in ovarian serous carcinoma and normal ovarian surface epithelium. *Cancer.* 2003;98(4):758–764.

82. Coleman RL, Broaddus RR, Bodurka DC, et al. Phase II trial of imatinib mesylate in patients with recurrent platinum- and taxane-resistant epithelial ovarian and primary peritoneal cancers. *Gynecol Oncol.* 2006;101(1):126–131.

83. Schilder RJ, Sill MW, Lee RB, et al. Phase II evaluation of imatinib mesylate in the treatment of recurrent or persistent epithelial ovarian or primary peritoneal carcinoma: A Gynecologic Oncology Group Study. *J Clin Oncol.* 2008;26(20):3418–3425.

84. Alberts DS, Liu PY, Wilczynski SP, et al. Phase II trial of imatinib mesylate in recurrent, biomarker positive, ovarian cancer (Southwest Oncology Group Protocol S0211). *Int J Gynecol Cancer.* 2007;17(4):784–788.

85. Posadas EM, Kwitkowski V, Kotz HL, et al. A prospective analysis of imatinib-induced c-KIT modulation in ovarian cancer: A phase II clinical study with proteomic profiling. *Cancer.* 2007;110(2):309–317.

86. Matei D, Emerson RE, Schilder J, et al. Imatinib mesylate in combination with docetaxel for the treatment of patients with advanced, platinum-resistant ovarian cancer and primary peritoneal carcinomatosis: A Hoosier Oncology Group trial. *Cancer.* 2008;113(4):723–732.

87. Taja-Chayeb L, Chavez-Blanco A, Martinez-Tlahuel J, et al. Expression of platelet derived growth factor family members and the potential role of imatinib mesylate for cervical cancer. *Cancer Cell Int.* 2006;6:22.

88. Candelaria M, Arias-Bonfill D, Chavez-Blanco A, et al. Lack in efficacy for imatinib mesylate as second-line treatment of recurrent or metastatic cervical cancer expressing platelet-derived growth factor receptor alpha. *Int J Gynecol Cancer.* 2009;19(9):1632–1637.

89. Wilhelm SM, Adnane L, Newell P, et al. Preclinical overview of sorafenib, a multikinase inhibitor that targets both Raf and VEGF and PDGF receptor tyrosine kinase signaling. *Mol Cancer Ther.* 2008;7(10):3129–3140.

90. Matei D, Sill MW, DeGeest K, Bristow RE. Phase II trial of sorafenib in persistent or recurrent epithelial ovarian cancer (EOC) or primary peritoneal cancer (PPC): A Gynecologic Oncology Group (GOG) study. *ASCO Meeting Abstracts.* 2008;26(15, suppl):5537.

91. Matei D, Ramasubbaiah R, Schilder J, et al. A phase I/II study of topotecan and sorafenib in recurrent, platinum-resistant ovarian cancer: HOG GYN-111. *ASCO Meeting Abstracts.* 2010;28(15, suppl):5108.

92. Hainsworth JD, Numnum TM, Rao GG. A randomized phase II study of paclitaxel/carboplatin with or without sorafenib in the first-line treatment of patients with stage III/IV epithelial ovarian cancer. *ASCO Meeting Abstracts.* 2010;28(15, suppl):TPS257.

93. Araujo J, Logothetis C. Dasatinib: A potent SRC inhibitor in clinical development for the treatment of solid tumors. *Cancer Treat Rev.* 2010;36(6):492–500.

94. Johnson FM, Agrawal S, Burris H, et al. Phase 1 pharmacokinetic and drug-interaction study of dasatinib in patients with advanced solid tumors. *Cancer.* 2010;116(6):1582–1591.

95. Morabito A, Piccirillo MC, Falasconi F, et al. Vandetanib (ZD6474), a dual inhibitor of vascular endothelial growth factor receptor (VEGFR) and epidermal growth factor receptor (EGFR) tyrosine kinases: Current status and future directions. *Oncologist.* 2009;14(4):378–390.

96. Annunziata CM, Walker AJ, Minasian L, et al. Vandetanib, designed to inhibit VEGFR2 and EGFR signaling, had no clinical activity as monotherapy for recurrent ovarian cancer and no detectable modulation of VEGFR2. *Clin Cancer Res.* 2010;16(2):664–672.

97. Chang F, Lee JT, Navolanic PM, et al. Involvement of PI3K/Akt pathway in cell cycle progression, apoptosis, and neoplastic transformation: a target for cancer chemotherapy. *Leukemia.* 2003;17(3):590–603.

98. Yuan ZQ, Sun M, Feldman RI, et al. Frequent activation of AKT2 and induction of apoptosis by inhibition of phosphoinositide-3-OH kinase/Akt pathway in human ovarian cancer. *Oncogene.* 2000;19(19):2324–2330.

99. Cristiano BE, Chan JC, Hannan KM, et al. A specific role for AKT3 in the genesis of ovarian cancer through modulation of G(2)-M phase transition. *Cancer Res.* 2006;66(24):11718–11725.

100. Zorn KK, Bonome T, Gangi L, et al. Gene expression profiles of serous, endometrioid, and clear cell subtypes of ovarian and endometrial cancer. *Clin Cancer Res.* 2005;11(18):6422–6430.

101. Liu Y, Xing H, Weng D, et al. Inhibition of Akt signaling by SN-38 induces apoptosis in cervical cancer. *Cancer Lett.* 2009;274(1):47–53.

102. Abe N, Watanabe J, Tsunoda S, et al. Significance of nuclear p-Akt in endometrial carcinogenesis: Rapid translocation of p-Akt Into the nucleus by estrogen, possibly resulting in inhibition of apoptosis. *Int J Gynecol Cancer.* 2011;21(2):194–202.

103. Rice LW, Stone RL, Xu M, et al. Biologic targets for therapeutic intervention in endometrioid endometrial adenocarcinoma and malignant mixed mullerian tumors. *Am J Obstet Gynecol.* 2006;194(4):1119–1126; discussion 1126–1128.

104. Mills GB, Fang X, Lu Y, et al. Specific keynote: Molecular therapeutics in ovarian cancer. *Gynecol Oncol.* 2003;88(1 Pt 2):S88–92; discussion S93–96.

105. Whitman M, Downes CP, Keeler M, et al. Type I phosphatidylinositol kinase makes a novel inositol phospholipid, phosphatidylinositol-3-phosphate. *Nature.* 1988;332(6165):644–646.

106. Walker EH, Pacold ME, Perisic O, et al. Structural determinants of phosphoinositide 3-kinase inhibition by wortmannin, LY294002, quercetin, myricetin, and staurosporine. *Mol Cell.* 2000;6(4):909–919.

107. Campbell IG, Russell SE, Choong DY, et al. Mutation of the PIK3CA gene in ovarian and breast cancer. *Cancer Res.* 2004;64(21):7678–7681.

108. Rudd ML, Price JC, Fogoros S, et al. A unique spectrum of somatic PIK3CA (p110alpha) mutations within primary endometrial carcinomas. *Clin Cancer Res.* 2011;17(6):1331–1340.

109. Urick ME, Rudd ML, Godwin AK, Sgroi D, Merino M, Bell DW. PIK3R1 (p85{alpha}) is somatically mutated at high frequency in primary endometrial cancer. *Cancer Res.* 2011;71(12):4061–4067.

110. Liu Y, Cui B, Qiao Y, et al. Phosphoinositide-3-kinase inhibition enhances radiosensitization of cervical cancer in vivo. *Int J Gynecol Cancer.* 2011;21(1):100–105.

111. Mutter GL, Lin MC, Fitzgerald JT, et al. Altered PTEN expression as a diagnostic marker for the earliest endometrial precancers. *J Natl Cancer Inst.* 2000;92(11):924–930.

112. Ji J, Zheng PS. Activation of mTOR signaling pathway contributes to survival of cervical cancer cells. *Gynecol Oncol.* 2010;117(1):103–108.

113. Mabuchi S, Altomare DA, Cheung M, et al. RAD001 inhibits human ovarian cancer cell proliferation, enhances cisplatin-induced apoptosis, and prolongs survival in an ovarian cancer model. *Clin Cancer Res.* 2007;13(14):4261–4270.

114. Mabuchi S, Kawase C, Altomare DA, et al. mTOR is a promising therapeutic target both in cisplatin-sensitive and cisplatin-resistant clear cell carcinoma of the ovary. *Clin Cancer Res.* 2009;15(17):5404–5413.

115. Miyazawa M, Yasuda M, Fujita M, et al. Therapeutic strategy targeting the mTOR-HIF-1alpha-VEGF pathway in ovarian clear cell adenocarcinoma. *Pathol Int.* 2009;59(1):19–27.

116. Kurose K, Zhou XP, Araki T, Cannistra SA, Maher ER, Eng C. Frequent loss of PTEN expression is linked to elevated phosphorylated Akt levels, but not associated with p27 and cyclin D1 expression, in primary epithelial ovarian carcinomas. *Am J Pathol.* 2001;158(6):2097–2106.

117. Zhu X, Kwon CH, Schlosshauer PW, et al. PTEN induces G(1) cell cycle arrest and decreases cyclin

D3 levels in endometrial carcinoma cells. *Cancer Res.* 2001;61(11):4569–4575.

118. Oda K, Stokoe D, Taketani Y, et al. High frequency of coexistent mutations of PIK3CA and PTEN genes in endometrial carcinoma. *Cancer Res.* 2005;65(23):10669–10673.

119. Oza AM, Elit L, Biagi J, et al. Molecular correlates associated with a phase II study of temsirolimus (CCI-779) in patients with metastatic or recurrent endometrial cancer—NCIC IND 160. *ASCO Meeting Abstracts.* 2006;24(18, suppl):3003.

120. Slomovitz BM, Lu KH, Johnston T, et al. A phase 2 study of the oral mammalian target of rapamycin inhibitor, everolimus, in patients with recurrent endometrial carcinoma. *Cancer.* 2010;116(23):5415–5419.

121. Slomovitz BM, Lu KH, Johnston T, et al. A phase II study of oral mammalian target of rapamycin (mTOR) inhibitor, RAD001 (everolimus), in patients with recurrent endometrial carcinoma (EC). *ASCO Meeting Abstracts.* 2008;26(15, suppl):5502.

122. Colombo N, McMeekin S, Schwartz P, et al. A phase II trial of the mTOR inhibitor AP23573 as a single agent in advanced endometrial cancer. *ASCO Meeting Abstracts.* 2007;25(18, suppl):5516.

123. Martin L, Schilder R. Novel approaches in advancing the treatment of epithelial ovarian cancer: The role of angiogenesis inhibition. *J Clin Oncol.* 2007;25(20):2894–2901.

124. Oza AM, Kollmannsberger C, NCIC Clinical Trials Group, et al. Phase I study of temsirolimus (CCI-779), carboplatin, and paclitaxel in patients (pts) with advanced solid tumors: NCIC CTG IND 179. *ASCO Meeting Abstracts.* 2009;27(15S):3558.

125. Dar AA, Goff LW, Majid S, et al. Aurora kinase inhibitors—rising stars in cancer therapeutics? *Mol Cancer Ther.* 2010;9(2):268–278.

126. Tao X, Chon HS, Fu S, et al. Update on aurora kinase inhibitors in gynecologic malignancies. *Recent Pat Anticancer Drug Discov.* 2008;3(3):162–177.

127. Campos SM, Ghosh S. A current review of targeted therapeutics for ovarian cancer. *J Oncol.* 2010;2010:149362.

128. Yang G, Chang B, Yang F, et al. Aurora kinase A promotes ovarian tumorigenesis through dysregulation of the cell cycle and suppression of BRCA2. *Clin Cancer Res.* 2010;16(12):3171–3181.

129. Mukhopadhyay A, Curtin N, Plummer R, et al. PARP inhibitors and epithelial ovarian cancer: An approach to targeted chemotherapy and personalised medicine. *BJOG.* 2011;118(4):429–432.

130. Press JZ, De Luca A, Boyd N, et al. Ovarian carcinomas with genetic and epigenetic BRCA1 loss have distinct molecular abnormalities. *BMC Cancer.* 2008;8:17.

131. Turner N, Tutt A, Ashworth A. Hallmarks of 'BRCAness' in sporadic cancers. *Nat Rev Cancer.* 2004;4(10):814–819.

132. Hughes-Davies L, Huntsman D, Ruas M, et al. EMSY links the BRCA2 pathway to sporadic breast and ovarian cancer. *Cell.* 2003;115(5):523–535.

133. Ashworth A. A synthetic lethal therapeutic approach: Poly(ADP) ribose polymerase inhibitors for the treatment of cancers deficient in DNA double-strand break repair. *J Clin Oncol.* 2008;26(22):3785–3790.

134. Audeh MW, Carmichael J, Penson RT, et al. Oral poly(ADP-ribose) polymerase inhibitor olaparib in patients with BRCA1 or BRCA2 mutations and recurrent ovarian cancer: A proof-of-concept trial. *Lancet.* 2010;376(9737):245–251.

135. Gelmon KA, Hirte HW, Robidoux A, et al. Can we define tumors that will respond to PARP inhibitors? A phase II correlative study of olaparib in advanced serous ovarian cancer and triple-negative breast cancer. *ASCO Meeting Abstracts.* 2010;28(15, suppl):3002.

136. Liu J, Fleming GF, Tolaney SM, et al. A phase I trial of the PARP inhibitor olaparib (AZD2281) in combination with the antiangiogenic cediranib (AZD2171) in recurrent ovarian or triple-negative breast cancer. *ASCO Meeting Abstracts.* 2011;29(15, suppl):5028.

137. Lee J, Annunziata CM, Minasian LM, et al. Phase I study of the PARP inhibitor olaparib (O) in combination with carboplatin (C) in BRCA1/2 mutation carriers with breast (Br) or ovarian (Ov) cancer (Ca). *ASCO Meeting Abstracts.* 2011;29(15, suppl):2520.

138. Liao X, Siu MK, Au CW, et al. Aberrant activation of hedgehog signaling pathway in ovarian cancers: Effect on prognosis, cell invasion and differentiation. *Carcinogenesis.* 2009;30(1):131–140.

139. Bhattacharya R, Kwon J, Ali B, et al. Role of hedgehog signaling in ovarian cancer. *Clin Cancer Res.* 2008;14(23):7659–7666.

140. Rueda BR, McCann C, Growdon WB, et al. Significance of the hedgehog (Hh) pathway in ovarian cancer xenograft growth. *ASCO Meeting Abstracts.* 2010;28(15, suppl):5058.

141. Berek JS, Schultes BC, Nicodemus CF. Biologic and immunologic therapies for ovarian cancer. *J Clin Oncol.* 2003;21(10 Suppl):168s–174s.

142. Liu B, Nash J, Runowicz C, Swede H, Stevens R, Li Z. Ovarian cancer immunotherapy: Opportunities, progresses and challenges. *J Hematol Oncol.* 2010;3:7.

143. Kandalaft LE, Powell DJ, Jr., Singh N, et al. Immunotherapy for ovarian cancer: W next? *J Clin Oncol.* 2011;29(7):925–933.

144. Sabbatini P, Odunsi K. Immunologic approaches to ovarian cancer treatment. *J Clin Oncol.* 2007;25(20):2884–2893.

145. Dougan M, Dranoff G. Immune therapy for cancer. *Annu Rev Immunol.* 2009;27:83–117.

146. Reichert JM. Antibody-based therapeutics to watch in 2011. *MAbs.* 2011;3(1):76–99.

147. Toffoli G, Cernigoi C, Russo A, et al. Overexpression of folate binding protein in ovarian cancers. *Int J Cancer.* 1997;74(2):193–198.

148. Konner JA, Bell-McGuinn KM, Sabbatini P, et al. Farletuzumab, a humanized monoclonal antibody against folate receptor alpha, in epithelial ovarian cancer: A phase I study. *Clin Cancer Res.* 2010;16(21): 5288–5295.

149. White AJ, Coleman RL, Armstrong DK, et al. Efficacy and safety of farletuzumab, a humanized monoclonal antibody to folate receptor alpha, in platinum-sensitive relapsed ovarian cancer subjects: Final data from a multicenter phase II study. *ASCO Meeting Abstracts.* 2010;28(15, suppl):5001.

150. Rosenberg SA, Lotze MT, Muul LM, et al. Observations on the systemic administration of autologous lymphokine-activated killer cells and recombinant interleukin-2 to patients with metastatic cancer. *N Engl J Med.* 1985;313(23):1485–1492.

151. Steis RG, Urba WJ, VanderMolen LA, et al. Intraperitoneal lymphokine-activated killer-cell and interleukin-2 therapy for malignancies limited to the peritoneal cavity. *J Clin Oncol.* 1990;8(10): 1618–1629.

152. West WH, Tauer KW, Yannelli JR, et al. Constant-infusion recombinant interleukin-2 in adoptive immunotherapy of advanced cancer. *N Engl J Med.* 1987;316(15):898–905.

153. Topalian SL, Solomon D, Avis FP, et al. Immunotherapy of patients with advanced cancer using tumor-infiltrating lymphocytes and recombinant interleukin-2: A pilot study. *J Clin Oncol.* 1988;6(5):839–853.

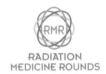

Lymphadenectomy in Uterine Cancer

Elizabeth Kathleen Nugent and Donald Scott McMeekin*

Department of Obstetrics and Gynecology, University of Oklahoma Health Science Center, Oklahoma, OK

■ ABSTRACT

Surgery is the mainstay of therapy for endometrial cancer, the most common type of gynecologic cancer. Evolution of surgical management has included the integration of lymph node assessment into the treatment of patients with endometrial cancer to better identify extent of disease, define prognosis, and tailor use of postoperative therapies. Strategies to identify the roughly 10% of patients with node-positive disease include routine versus selective use of lymphadenectomy. Data from prospective and retrospective series offer conflicting opinions on the routine use of nodal dissections. In this review, which patients to consider for lymphadenectomy, the extent of surgery, and surgical techniques are discussed. The downstream consequences of caring for women with endometrial cancer where nodal status is known or unknown must also be considered. In addition, complications and sequelae of lymphadenectomy should be balanced by the information obtained.

Keywords: endometrial cancer, lymphadenectomy

■ INTRODUCTION

Endometrial cancer accounts for >50% of all new gynecologic cancers diagnosed in the United States, representing the fourth most common malignancy in women and the eighth most common cause of cancer death. The American Cancer Society estimated 43,470 new cases of endometrial carcinoma and 7,950 deaths from disease in 2010 (1). Endometrial cancer is commonly confined to the uterus at diagnosis. Data from the National Cancer Institute's Surveillance, Epidemiology, and End Results (SEER) program and the 26th Annual Report of the International Federation of Gynecology and Obstetrics (FIGO) demonstrated that 83% of patients were diagnosed with early stage (stage I–II) disease (2,3). Along with favorable disease distribution at presentation, most patients have favorable prognosis. Results from the FIGO reveal that 85% to 91% of stage I patients are alive at 5 years, and patients in the SEER database with localized disease have a 96% survival at 5 years (2,3). Despite the favorable characteristics for a majority of patients, those with high-risk factors including increased age, high tumor grade, aggressive histology, and advanced stage face significant challenges.

Of all the female pelvic malignancies, endometrial cancer seems to have more advocates for different

*Corresponding author, Division of Gynecologic Oncology, University of Oklahoma Health Science Center, P.O. Box 26901, WP 2410, Oklahoma City, OK 73126
E-mail address: scott-mcmeekin@ouhsc.edu

Radiation Medicine Rounds 2:3 (2011) 425–438.
DOI: 10.5003/2151–4208.2.3.425

treatment approaches than any other. Standard treatment has been and remains a hysterectomy. However, through the years, preoperative and postoperative radiation have had important roles in the management of this disease. The first significant report of employing radiation in the management of women with endometrial cancer was the "Stockholm Technique" by Heyman in 1935 using a single intrauterine tandem (4). The use of single-tandem implants transitioned to the use of multiple intrauterine capsules, which were associated with a lower incidence of residual disease and an improved 5-year survival rate (5–7). By the 1960s, endometrial cancer patients were frequently managed with preoperative pelvic radiation therapy (RT), low dose rate (LDR) brachytherapy with or without pelvic RT followed up within 4 to 6 weeks by a completion hysterectomy. Surgical evaluation of lymph nodes in endometrial cancer was also reported in the 1960s, but not widely embraced (8–11). In an era where essentially all patients received pelvic RT, nodal status was, perhaps, irrelevant.

In 1987, the Gynecologic Oncology Group (GOG) reported a large surgical-pathologic study of clinical stage I endometrial cancer patients (GOG 33), which better defined patterns of spread and identified pathologic relationships between uterine characteristics and nodal disease (12,13). This study helped lead to a tailored approach to RT and to an adoption of a surgical staging system for endometrial cancer in 1988. The surgical management of women with endometrial cancer has further evolved to include more common use of pelvic and paraaortic lymphadenectomy, introduction and acceptance of minimally invasive surgery (laparoscopic and robotic), and the evaluation of sentinel mapping techniques. Increased use of surgical staging has translated to less frequent use of RT and particularly a reduction whole pelvic irradiation (12). Important developments in combination chemotherapy have also occurred with chemotherapy increasingly used in the recurrent and adjuvant settings.

■ IMPORTANCE OF AND ALTERNATIVES TO LYMPHADENECTOMY

A better understanding of the natural history of endometrial cancer has resulted from the systematic evaluation of patterns of spread in the GOG 33 study (13). This trial included 621 patients with clinical stage I or occult stage II endometrial cancer undergoing a standardized surgical procedure (exploration of the abdomen, biopsy of suspicious findings, collection of peritoneal fluid, abdominal hysterectomy, bilateral salpingo-oophorectomy, and pelvic and paraaortic nodal dissection). Overall, 22% of patients with seemingly uterine-confined disease were found to have extrauterine spread. Pelvic nodal metastases were documented in 9% of patients, paraaortic disease in 5%, 12% had positive peritoneal cytology, 5% had adnexal involvement, and 6% had gross intraperitoneal spread. Nodal metastases were associated with increasing tumor grade and deeper myometrial invasion, and patients with positive cytology, adnexal, or intraperitoneal spread also had increased frequency of nodal disease. In GOG 33, extent of disease found at surgery was predictive of patient outcomes, demonstrating the important relationship between surgical findings and recurrence risk (14).

Importance of Stage

Stage is used to categorize patients into high- and low-risk groups and to guide the use of adjuvant therapies. The prognostic utility of surgicopathologic stage has been confirmed in multiple studies (13,15–22). In 2009, FIGO staging for endometrial cancer was revised (Table 1). Retrospective comparison of clinical and surgicopathologic staging demonstrated superiority of surgicopathologic staging in predicting outcomes and surgical stage is often the single strongest predictor of outcome for women with endometrial adenocarcinoma (15). Patients with nodal metastases (stage IIIC) disease have a poorer prognosis compared with node-negative populations. FIGO data show 5-year survival to be 57% in stage IIIC patients compared with 74% to 91% when nodes are negative (stage I–II). Patients with positive pelvic but negative paraaortic nodes also have a better prognosis compared with those with paraaortic disease involvement (14,23). Two retrospective series have also suggested that patients with nodal disease in addition to positive cytology, adnexa, or serosa extension have poorer progression-free survival (PFS) or overall survival compared with patients with positive nodes alone (23,24). Lymphadenectomy (25–27), complete surgical resection of bulky nodes (28), and the use of chemotherapy (29–31) have been suggested to improve outcomes in patients and modify the prognostic effect of nodal disease.

TABLE 1   2009 FIGO staging system for carcinoma of the endometrium

Stage I[a]		Tumor contained to the corpus uteri
	IA	No or less than half myometrial invasion
	IB	Invasion equal to or more than half of the myometrium
Stage II		Tumor invades the cervical stroma but does not extend beyond the uterus[b]
Stage II[a]		Local and/or regional spread of tumor[c]
	IIIA	Tumor invades the serosa of the corpus uteri and/or adnexas
	IIIB	Vaginal and/or parametrial involvement
	IIIC	Metastases to pelvis and/or paraaortic lymph nodes
		IIIC1 Positive pelvic nodes
		IIIC2 Positive para-aortic lymph nodes with or without positive pelvic lymph nodes
Stage IV[a]		Tumor invades bladder and/or bowel mucosa and/or distant metastases
	IVA	Tumor invasion of bladder and/or bowel mucosa
	IVB	Distant metastases, including intra-abdominal metastases and or inguinal lymph nodes

[a]Includes grades 1, 2, or 3.
[b]Endocervical glandular involvement only should be considered as stage I and no longer as stage II.
[c]Positive cytology has to be reported separately without changing the stage.

Preoperative Imaging and Biopsy

Preoperative imaging and biopsy specimens as surrogates for staging have been studied extensively, but remain an inadequate measure of overall disease extent found at surgical exploration. For example, Ben-Shachar et al. and Goudge et al. compared endometrial sampling and final uterine pathology and determined that about 20% of tumors were upgraded (32,33). Various imaging modalities have been examined preoperatively to assess uterine factors and lymph node status in patients with endometrial cancer. Computed tomography (CT) scans have lower sensitivity than magnetic resonance imaging (MRI), which has a staging accuracy of about 85%. MRI has only a 54% sensitivity in determining uterine factors such as myometrial invasion and a sensitivity of 45% in detection of lymph node metastases (34,35). Selman and colleagues preformed a systematic literature review of tests for lymph node status and suggested that MRI appeared to be superior to CT evaluations (35). Positron emission tomography (PET)/CT has also been utilized to detect lymph node involvement with a sensitivity of approximately 67%, which is comparable to MRI (36,37).

Intraoperative Evaluation

Intraoperative evaluation, including lymph node palpation and frozen sectioning of the uterus during surgery, has been used to determine which patients should undergo complete surgical staging. Unfortunately, both methods of intraoperative assessment are associated with poor reproducibility and inaccurate prediction of extrauterine disease involvement. Lymph node palpation is often inaccurate because micro-metastasis of carcinoma to nodes is the most common finding. Of positive lymph nodes examined, 13% to 40% of lymph node metastasis were reported as <2 mm and only 7% to 10% of lymph nodes were grossly enlarged (≥2 cm) (38,39). Lymph node palpation has a 26% to 36% false-negative rate in large cohorts of patients with gynecologic malignancies (40–42). Intraoperative uterine examination with frozen section has varying success in predicting final pathological diagnosis and stage of disease. Frozen section may lead to under appreciation of depth of invasion or tumor grade in about 15% to 20% of cases.

Uterine Factors as a Surrogate to Predict Nodal Disease

In patients who do not undergo a nodal dissection at the time of hysterectomy, final pathological information identifying particular uterine risk factors can be used to estimate the risk of nodal involvement and aid in decisions to offer adjuvant RT. In GOG 33, pelvic and paraaortic nodal disease was more frequent with increasing grade (percentage of pelvic nodal metastases: 3% grade I, 9% grade II, and 18% grade 3), depth of invasion (1% endometrium only, 5% inner one-third, 6% middle one-third, and 25% outer one-third myometrial invasion), and lymphovascular space invasion (LVSI) (27% with LVSI and 7% without LVSI) (13) (Table 2). Patients with disease of the lower uterine segment also have a higher incidence of pelvic and paraaortic lymph node metastases (16%) than do those with fundal-only disease (8% and 4%, respectively). Despite the use of uterine pathology to help predict nodal disease, many believe that routine lymph node assessment is superior as it provides actual information on nodal status, as opposed to an estimate, which can then be used to tailor adjuvant therapies.

■ THE CONTROVERSY

In terms of nodal assessment of disease, large prospective trials demonstrate that nodal metastases in women presenting with clinically uterine-confined disease occurs in ~10% of patients (Table 3). The extent which nodal disease effects prognosis and alters the use of postoperative therapies is clear. Surgeons are challenged with distinguishing those relatively few patients with nodal disease from the larger population without disease. Current clinical controversies center on the extent of nodal surgery, selection of which patients to offer dissection, and what to do with the information obtained. For example, Kwon and colleagues evaluated a population-based cohort study including 316 surgically staged patients and found that pelvic nodal status was not an independent predictor of survival (42). Uterine characteristics such as grade 3 tumors, deep invasion, and cervical involvement were more important determinants of survival. In addition, the GOG 99 trial (prospective randomized trial of pelvic RT versus observation in patients with node-negative disease) demonstrated that even in the setting of negative nodes, 27% of patients with high-risk uterine features recurred (43).

TABLE 2   Frequency of nodal metastases based on pathologic risk factors in GOG 33

Risk Factor	Frequency of Nodal Metastasis		
	No. of Patients	Pelvic No. (%)	Aortic No. (%)
Histology			
Endometrioid adenocarcinoma	599	56 (9)	30 (5)
Others	22	2 (9)	4 (18)
Grade			
1 Well	180	5 (3)	3 (2)
2 Moderate	288	25 (9)	14 (5)
3 Poor	153	28 (18)	17 (11)
Myometrial invasion			
Endometrial	87	1 (1)	1 (1)
Superficial	279	15 (5)	8 (3)
Middle	116	7 (6)	1 (1)
Deep	139	35 (25)	24 (17)
Site of tumor location			
Fundus	524	42 (8)	20 (4)
Isthmus-cervix	97	16 (16)	14 (14)
Capillary-like space involvement			
Negative	528	37 (7)	19 (9)
Positive	93	21 (27)	15 (19)
Other extrauterine metastasis			
Negative	586	40 (7)	26 (4)
Positive	35	18 (51)	8 (23)
Peritoneal cytology[a]			
Negative	537	38 (7)	20 (4)
Positive	75	19 (25)	14 (19)

[a]Nine patients did not have cytology reported.
Modified from Ref. (41)

TABLE 3 Frequency of nodal metastases in patients with clinically early-stage endometrial cancer

Study	*n*	Frequency of Nodal Disease
GOG 33 (13)	621	9%
ASTEC (lymphadenectomy arm) (29)	686	9%
Benedetti (lymphadenectomy arm) (51)	264	13%
LAP II (71)	2510	9%
ASTEC (no lymphadenectomy arm) (29)	685	1%
Benedetti (no lymphadenectomy arm) (51)	250	3%

These data do not downplay the clinical significance of nodal disease, but highlight the fact that recurrence and survival may be impacted by factors in addition to nodal status.

Fundamentally, surgeons must determine whether or not they believe that surgical staging has sufficient value to offer it to all patients or only selectively based on risk factors identified pre- and intraoperatively. Questions relate to which patients should be offered and could benefit from surgical staging (all, some, none), and what is the optimal surgical procedure to be performed (biopsy of enlarged/visible nodes, lymphadenectomy). Controversy also exists between surgeons who perform only pelvic dissections and those who advocate pelvic and paraaortic nodal dissection. If paraaortic nodes are removed, are bilateral nodes required, and to what superior extent (inferior mesenteric artery, renal vessels) should the dissection proceed? If a patient is not offered surgical staging/nodal dissection, then minimizing surgical morbidity with a vaginal or laparoscopic-assisted approach may be warranted.

Nodal Dissection—None

In the United States, comprehensive surgical staging of endometrial cancer is infrequently performed with only 30% to 40% of patients undergoing nodal assessment (43,44). Most gynecologists are not trained to perform lymphadenectomy and full staging is more commonly performed by gynecologic oncologists. Philosophically, those opposed to nodal dissections suggest that most patients are at low risk for nodal disease, treatment decisions can be based on final pathologic information, and despite node dissection the majority of patients who are node negative do not benefit (45). The Post Operative Radiation Therapy in Endometrial Cancer (PORTEC) trial evaluated women with stage IC grade 1, stage IB-C grade 2,

or stage IB grade 3 who underwent hysterectomy without lymph node dissection and compared observation to postoperative pelvic RT (46). This patient population managed without nodal dissection and had favorable outcomes with or without RT (5-year survival rates of 85% observation, 81% with pelvic irradiation). Trimble et al. reported on a cohort of stage I endometrial cancer patients collected by SEER from 1988 to 1993 and showed 5-year relative survival for patients without nodal dissection was 98% compared with 96% in those undergoing nodal dissection, suggesting that nodal dissection did not convey a benefit for the overall population (47). In a nonrandomized trial comparing hysterectomy with or without pelvic lymphadenectomy, followed by RT, 14% of patients (*n* = 207) with negative nodes treated with vaginal cuff brachytherapy recurred compared with 16% who did not have a lymphadenectomy (*n* = 660) (48). While the authors noted similar cancer-free survival between the two groups, all patients who did not have nodal dissections received both pelvic RT and vaginal brachytherapy to attain these results. It is suspected that the increased use of RT in unstaged patients may produce similar outcomes to patients who are surgically staged who avoid RT.

Two recent large randomized trials comparing lymphadenectomy to no nodal assessment have been recently published and have increased the debate on the value of lymphadenectomy. A Study in the Treatment of Endometrial Cancer (ASTEC) randomized 1,408 women with endometrial cancer to hysterectomy with and without pelvic lymphadenectomy. Following surgery, patients with early-stage disease at intermediate risk of recurrence (*n* = 905) were randomized independent of nodal status to observation or pelvic RT. Interestingly, vaginal cuff brachytherapy could be used regardless of radiation randomization or lymphadenectomy (49,50). Results of the surgical portion of the trial suggested no advantage of routine lymphadenectomy in terms of recurrence or overall survival. Of note, patients who underwent routine lymphadenectomy more commonly were identified with node-positive disease (9%) compared with patients who did not undergo routine staging (1%). In addition, postoperative complications or adverse events were more common following lymphadenectomy. An Italian trial randomized 514 patients with FIGO stage I endometrial cancer to surgery with or without systematic pelvic lymphadenectomy (51). The use of postoperative therapy was at the discretion of the treating physician. Both early and late surgical complications occurred more frequently in women receiving pelvic lymphadenectomy. Pelvic lymphadenectomy improved surgical staging accuracy with identification of more patients with lymph node metastasis in the group undergoing lymphadenectomy (13% vs. 3%, $p < .001$), but no significant difference in overall survival or PFS was noted between the arms. Of note, patients who did not undergo lymphadenectomy more commonly received pelvic RT postoperatively.

A great deal discussion about these trials has occurred in the literature since their publication (54,55). One concern is that for nodal dissection to be of value, a representative resection of nodes at risk must be performed. In both trials, the adequacy of lymph node dissection is in question. In the ASTEC trial, greater than a third of the women in the "node dissection" group had nine or fewer lymph nodes removed. Neither trial required paraaortic lymph node dissection. In a recent retrospective analysis from Japan, Todo and colleagues showed that in patients managed with systematic pelvic and paraaortic lymphadenectomy, survival was improved compared with patients managed with pelvic lymphadenectomy only (hazard ratio 0.53, $p = .005$) (56). As >50% of node-positive patients have paraaortic involvement, the lack of paraaortic nodal evaluation may alter outcomes. The potential adjuvant treatment may also compromise the ability of nodal dissection to demonstrate improvements. For example, if patients without nodal dissection received postoperative therapy more commonly, then could radiation mask the lack of nodal dissection? Both the ASTEC and Italian studies have been criticized by the inclusion of a relatively low risk group of patients. For example, only 106 node-positive patients were included in the trials such that there was low power to see difference in outcomes particularly in women likely to benefit from nodal dissection (i.e., node-positive patients). Some have suggested that enrichment with

higher-risk patients would be required for an possible advantage of lymphadenectomy to be identified. Although both the ASTEC study and the Italian trial suggest no benefit to lymph node dissection, by no means has this argument been put to rest.

If physicians do not obtain nodal information, they must rely on uterine factors to estimate the probability for nodal disease determine postoperative radiation necessity. This estimation can result in a substantial increase in the use of radiation and may also lead to poorer outcomes. In one study, patients with stage IC, grade 3 endometrial cancer without lymph node dissection were treated with pelvic RT and followed prospectively (52). Five-year survival was 58% and 12% had vaginal or pelvic failures despite pelvic radiation RT, a poorer outcome than stage IIIC patients managed by lymphadenectomy followed by RT (24,27,53).

Nodal Dissection—Selective

Since its incorporation into the staging of endometrial cancer in 1988, nodal assessment has been increasingly integrated into management. Many believe nodal dissection should be reserved for those with sufficient risk of nodal disease (13,14,54,55). At what risk of nodal disease (3, 5, 10% etc.) warrants the procedure is a matter of debate. Some investigators advocate that lymph nodes need not be sampled for tumor limited to the endometrium, regardless of grade, because >1% of these patients have disease spread to pelvic or paraaortic lymph nodes (13,56). Patients with serous or clear cell histology warrant nodal dissection as about 30% to 50% will have nodal disease, and even in the absence of myometrial invasion, nodal metastases have been reported in up to 36% of these patients (57). Investigators at the Mayo clinic have suggested that in patients with grade 1 or 2 tumor, myometrial invasion ≤50%, and tumor diameter ≤2 cm, lymph node dissection may be safely omitted. And in their series, no patients had positive lymph nodes or died of disease (41,62). The infrequency of nodal metastases in patients using the Mayo criteria was confirmed on retrospective examination of a large cohort of patients, demonstrating a 1% rate of nodal metastasis in those qualifying as low risk disease (63).

An assessment of both pelvic and paraaortic lymph nodes is required to assign stage. In GOG 33, the rate of paraaortic nodal involvement was roughly

50% of the pelvic nodal rate and isolated positive paraaortic nodes occurred in only 2% of cases. About half of positive paraaortic lymph nodes were found to be enlarged at the time of surgery and 98% of paraaortic node metastases were in those with positive pelvic nodes, adnexal or intraabdominal metastases, or outer one-third myometrial invasion (14). Paraaortic nodal dissection is more difficult to perform than pelvic dissection, by laparotomy or by laparoscopy, and is associated with greater risk. As such, some investigators advocate for pelvic nodal dissections with only performing paraaortic nodal dissections selectively.

Nodal Dissection—Routine

Many gynecologic oncologists have moved toward performing routine comprehensive surgical staging for nearly all patients with endometrial cancer. Surveys of gyn-oncology professional societies suggest that 75% to 90% routinely perform lymphadenectomy. The rationale for routine staging include the lack of a patient population for whom nodal disease is so low that nodes should be omitted, the inaccuracy of preoperative or intraoperative assessments predicting the risk for nodal disease, the potential for therapeutic benefit in node-positive and -negative patients, and the lack of significant morbidity associated with the procedure. Moving from a sampling technique to a more thorough lymphadenectomy is not associated with increased complication rates (58). Nodal dissection should be bilateral given the frequency of both left and right paraaortic involvement (59,60). Postoperative adjuvant therapy decisions are best made with the most complete information. If nodal assessment is the predominant factor by which to categorize patients into risk groups, routine nodal dissection is the best method by which to determine which few patients will require adjuvant therapy.

What constitutes an acceptable rate of nodal disease in endometrial cancer to warrant the procedure is surgeon dependent. In cervical cancer, routine pelvic lymphadenectomy is advocated for all stage IA2 tumors where nodal positivity rates are 3% to 5% (61). For clinical stage I ovarian cancer, paraaortic dissection is recommended for all patients given the 6% risk of paraaortic disease (62). In endometrial cancer, major complication rates associated with nodal dissection are 2% to 6% suggesting that this might be

an appropriate level of risk to balance against the risk of nodal metastases.

Extent of Nodal Dissection

The technique of nodal dissection has undergone evolution. In an era where all patients received RT, there was little value for a complete evaluation of lymph nodes. Today, adjuvant therapies are based on the extent of disease, and are often reserved for node-positive patients. If a full nodal assessment is performed, it should sufficiently examine external iliac, hypogastric, and obturator nodes in the pelvis, common iliac nodes, and paraaortic nodes superiorly. Nodal dissection is more apt to be representative when a larger number of nodes are removed.

The importance of paraaortic nodal spread in node-positive endometrial cancer cannot be ignored (Table 4). If the goal of nodal dissection is to identify the node-positive patient population, paraaortic disease is seen in 40% to 66% of patients with node-positive/stage IIIC endometrial cancer, including isolated positive paraaortic nodes in 7% to 21% of cases (12,27,28,66,69,72–74). If only pelvic nodes are removed, when they are positive, paraaortic nodes will be positive in addition in nearly 30 to 40% of cases. It thus makes little sense to remove only pelvic or only paraaortic nodes. Data also suggests when paraaortic lymph nodes are positive, outcomes are improved in patients who have complete surgical resection. Chuang et al. reported on selective pelvic and/or paraaortic dissections and found that failure to systematically remove lymph nodes resulted in an increased frequency of recurrence in undissected retroperitoneal sites (25). Similarly, Mariani and colleagues showed that patients at high risk for paraaortic nodal disease (based on myometrial invasion >50%, palpable positive pelvic nodes, positive adnexa) who did not undergo complete paraaortic dissection and were managed as though paraaortic nodes were positive had 5-year survival of 71% compared with 85% for those patients with positive paraaortic nodes who did undergo complete resection (58). Lymph node recurrences were detected in 37% of those not having paraaortic dissection compared with none in patients with positive but resected paraaortic nodes suggesting a possible therapeutic effect of removing involved paraaortic nodes. At the present time, the superior extent of paraaortic dissection is controversial. Some investigators suggest dissections should extend to

TABLE 4 Relationship between pelvic and para-aortic nodal involvement in patients with node-positive endometrial cancer

Study	n	Surgical Technique	Pelvic (+) Only (%)	Pelvic and Paraaortic (+) (%)	Paraaortic Only (%)	Any involvement of paraaortic nodes (%)
Creasman et al. (13)	70	Routine sampling	51	31	17	48
Schorge et al. (86)	35	Selective lymphadenectomy	74	17	9	26
Hirahatake et al. (63)	42	Routine systematic lymphadenectomy	57	38	5	42
Onda et al. (27)	30	Routine systematic lymphadenectomy	33	60	6.6	66
McMeekin et al. (60)	47	Routine lymphadenectomy	38	41	21	62
Otsuka et al. (87)	23	Selective systematic lymphadenectomy	66	33	10	43
Havrilesky et al. (28)	96	Selective lymphadenectomy	52	30	18	48

the level of the inferior mesenteric artery and others suggest dissection should proceed to the level of the renal vessels. In one series, 7 of 11 patients had positive paraaortic nodes identified above the inferior mesenteric artery (63). Prospective data describing the frequency of high paraaortic/ pararenal nodes are awaited.

No prospective data exist to adequately evaluate the claim that lymphadenectomy in endometrial cancer is therapeutic. The only prospective trial evaluating the role of lymphadenectomy (ASTEC trial) required only a pelvic lymphadenectomy and utilized a second randomization for pelvic radiation, which would typically be avoided after a negative lymphadenectomy (49,50), making results difficult to interpret. The available retrospective data suggesting a therapeutic benefit are largely from single institutions, have short follow-up, suffer from selection biases, and do not clearly account for stage migration.

Despite these limitations, Kilgore and colleagues were among the first to report a therapeutic effect of nodal dissections in a series of 649 clinical stage I, occult II patients (64). Patients who underwent multiple site pelvic nodal dissection (defined by dissection of at least four pelvic nodal sites) and had a mean of 11 nodes removed had improved survival over those patients who did not have nodes sampled. The survival advantage for multiple site dissection persisted when patients were stratified into uterus-confined

disease and extrauterine disease receiving radiation. Others have shown improvement in outcomes following a more complete nodal dissection in node-negative populations. Cragan et al. evaluated 509 stage I–IIa patients who underwent selective pelvic +/– paraaortic lymphadenectomy and found a survival advantage for patients with grade 3 tumors with >11 pelvic nodes removed compared with those with <11 nodes removed (hazard ratio 0.25) (65). For patients with high-risk features (grade 3, >50% myometrial invasion, serous/clear cell tumors), 5-year survival was 82% when >11 nodes were removed versus 64% when ≤ 11 nodes were removed. Chan and colleagues reported on the effect of a more complete nodal dissection in over 12,000 women with endometrial cancer tracked in the SEER data system (77). In patients with patients with high-risk disease (stages IB/grade 3, IC, II-IV), 5-year survival was proportional to the number of nodes removed increasing from 75% to 87% when 1 versus >20 nodes were removed. In a multivariate analysis, a more extensive nodal assessment was an independent predictor of survival.

In patients with positive pelvic and/or paraaortic nodes, complete nodal dissection followed by adjuvant therapy results in superior outcomes. Mariani et al. showed that pelvic side wall failure at 5 years was 57% for women who had inadequate nodal dissection and/or no adjuvant RT compared with 10% when patients had adequate (removal >10 nodes) lymphadenectomy and received RT (26). Patients with bulky residual nodes have a poorer survival compared with those who have the nodes successfully resected. The best outcomes reported for node-positive patients follow complete nodal dissection. In one series, 30 stage IIIC patients were managed with systematic pelvic and paraaortic lymphadenectomy (average number nodes removed, 66) followed by RT and chemotherapy and 5-year survival was 100% for patients with positive pelvic nodes and 75% for positive paraaortic nodes (27).

The most cogent argument for routine staging is following thorough nodal assessment, most patients with node-negative disease can accurately be classified as low risk and may avoid pelvic RT or receive vaginal cuff brachytherapy alone. Three randomized trials comparing pelvic irradiation to observation have failed to demonstrate a survival advantage for adjuvant pelvic RT in patients with stage I–II disease, suggesting that in the absence of nodal disease no therapy is a reasonable option (46,49,66). Retrospective studies have demonstrated incorporation of lymphadenectomy changes the use of postoperative RT (8,33,67–70). In the absence of nodal disease, recurrence risk is low and overall survival is high, with no pelvic RT or with the substitution of vaginal cuff brachytherapy.

■ LYMPHADENECTOMY TECHNIQUE

Surgical Technique

Contemporary surgical management for patients with endometrial cancer includes at the minimum, an initial surgical exploration with collection of peritoneal fluid for cytologic evaluation (intraperitoneal cell washings), thorough inspection of the abdominal and pelvic cavities with biopsy or excision of any extrauterine lesions suspicious for tumor, and total extrafascial hysterectomy with bilateral salpingo-oophorectomy. In cases of gross omental or intraperitoneal disease spread, cytoreductive surgery with total omentectomy, radical peritoneal stripping, and occasionally, bowel resection, are required. The goal of reducing the residual to no or small volumes akin to what is performed for ovarian cancer is increasingly considered.

When complete surgical staging is performed, the margins of the pelvic nodal dissection are comparable to what is used for a pelvic nodal dissection in cervical cancer and is outlined by the margins of

the circumflex iliac vein distally, the bifurcation of the iliac vessels proximally, the lateral margin is the genitofemoral nerve, and the medial margin is the superior vesical artery. The floor of the dissection is the obturator nerve. Nodal/fatty tissue is skeletonized from these structures. In cases of bulky nodal disease, complete resection/debulking rather than biopsy to solely demonstrate metastatic disease is favored whenever possible. The common iliac nodes can be removed as a separate specimen, or divided at a midpoint along the vessels, submitting the inferior half with the pelvic nodes, and the superior half with the paraaortic nodes. Particularly on the left side, the common iliac nodes will be quite lateral in location and will require sufficient mobilization to visualize the nodes. Removal of paraaortic nodes can be performed via a midline peritoneal incision over the common iliac arteries and aorta or by mobilizing the right and left colon medially. In each case, lymph nodes are resected along the upper common iliac vessels on either side and from the lower portion of the aorta and vena cava. The inferior mesenteric artery is generally used to demarcate the superior extent of the paraaortic nodal dissection, but suspicious nodes extending to the renal vessels should also be removed.

Minimally Invasive Management

While the tradition has been to perform this surgery abdominally (typically through a vertical midline incision), laparoscopic management has increasingly been integrated into practice. Laparoscopic techniques are utilized in the initial treatment of endometrial cancer as well as to restage patients following incomplete surgical staging. Laparoscopic techniques and tools making comprehensive surgical staging of endometrial cancer possible were introduced in the 1990s and computer-assisted laparoscopic surgery was approved by the Food and Drug Administration (FDA) in 2005. Multiple features of the robotic surgical platform make it ideally suited to complex surgery routinely performed by gynecologic oncologists. A multi-institutional randomized controlled trial performed by the GOG, LAP II, demonstrated feasibility of laparoscopic surgery with similar number of nodes removed, similar frequency of nodal positivity, and similar complication rates between open and laparoscopic surgery (71).

Compared with open procedures, laparoscopic-assisted vaginal hysterectomy and total laparoscopic hysterectomy (LAVH/TLH) are thought to lead to reduced blood loss intraoperatively, and postoperatively reduced incisional complications, wound infections, ileus, hospital stay, cost, and improve rate of recovery and quality of life (71–73). In patients requiring postoperative RT, laparoscopic surgical staging followed by RT is suggested to result in fewer bowel adhesions and radiation-induced bowel injuries (74). Criticisms of LAVH/TLH with laparoscopic nodal dissection relate to the learning curve required to learn new or unfamiliar procedures, the increased length of operative times, and concerns about the adequacy of nodal dissection. Laparoscopy also introduced different procedural-related complications. For example, it has the potential to produce port-site recurrences or intraperitoneal dissemination of disease by laparoscopic gas and/or uterine manipulation, although the frequency of these events is rare. Results of long-term survival in laparoscopically and robotically treated endometrial cancer patients are still limited.

Multi-institutional comparisons between traditional laparoscopic surgery and robotic surgery in staging of endometrial cancer have been published indicating further reduction in blood loss and hospital stay with the use of robotic surgery and a lower rate of conversion to open procedures (75–79). Complications and nodal yield do not appear to significantly differ between minimally invasive methods, but longer operative time is common in patients undergoing robotic surgery. In the subset of morbidly obese patients, robotic surgery seems to be associated with improvements in operative time and nodal yield.

One of the more useful roles of laparoscopic surgery is in the restaging of patients who underwent hysterectomy only. Patients who undergo hysterectomy without nodal dissection and who have pathologic risk factors for potential nodal spread face a difficult dilemma. Such patients may elect to receive RT or chemotherapy (presume nodes are positive), elect observation (presume nodes are negative), or undergo a second operation. A second laparotomy can be difficult to accept. Laparoscopic staging offers the patient a less invasive option to collect information.

Whether a LAVH/TLH or robotic procedure is comparable with an open approach must be individually judged by the ability to accurately dissect appropriate nodal basins, to remove an adequate/representative number of lymph nodes, to identify metastatic disease, and by the rates of recurrence.

Despite the potential benefits of laparoscopic surgery, if laparoscopic nodal dissection cannot be performed, conversion to laparotomy is advised when incomplete staging results would yield inadequate information for treatment planning. Demonstration of comparable surgical endpoints (similar numbers of nodes removed, similar frequency of positive nodes) along with shortened hospital stay and quicker recovery compared with open procedures suggests laparoscopic and robotic surgical staging is an excellent option in appropriate patients.

Another option for gaining information about nodal status is sentinel lymph node dissection, the standard of care in breast cancer and melanoma, which is gaining popularity in gynecologic malignancies. Retrospective reviews of sentinel lymph node dissection report a detection rate of 73% to 94% depending on experience with the procedure and a false-negative rate approaching zero (80,81). The SENTI-ENDO trial, a prospective European multicenter study of 133 patients undergoing cervical injection with blue dye and technetium in patients with endometrial cancer, reported a negative predictive value of 97%, a sensitivity of 84%, and concluded the technique represents a reasonable alternative to systematic lymphadenectomy (82). Advocates of sentinel dissection suggest the technique may reduce the need for complete lymphadenectomy and reduce postoperative complications such as lymphedema.

■ COMPLICATIONS ASSOCIATED WITH LYMPHADENECTOMY

In cases where nodal dissection will or potentially will be performed, patients must be adequately counseled regarding the risks and benefits. The principle risks attributable to nodal dissections include increased operative time, potential for blood loss associated with vascular injury, genitofemoral nerve injury with resulting numbness and paresthesia over the medial thighs, lymphocyst formation, and lymphedema (14,69,83,84) (Table 5). The overall surgical complication rate after lymphadenectomy is about 20% with a serious complication rate of ≤6%. Lymphedema is an underrecognized and underreported complication with estimates of 10% to 15% (64). Patients who have nodal dissections and receive pelvic RT may be at a greater risk of bowel morbidity than those without dissections (66,85). Many believe the rate of complications should be balanced by the probability of

TABLE 5 Risks associated with nodal dissection: Surgical complication rates associated with abdominal hysterectomy + pelvic and para-aortic lymph node dissection

Study	*n*	Hemorrhage (%)	GU Injury (%)	DVT/PE (%)	Lymphocyst (%)	Other
Morrow et al. (14)	895	2.2	0.4	2	1.2	
Homesley et al. (84)	196	6% transfused	–	4	–	"Serious" 6%
Orr et al. (69)	396	4.2% transfused	0.6	1.5	1.2	
Mariani et al. (26)	96 Node (+) pts	–	1	1	3.1	

DVT, deep venous thrombosis; PE, pulmonary embolus.

finding nodal disease and by the associated reduction in use of postoperative pelvic RT. In general, the risks associated with nodal dissections are low and acceptable. Nodal dissections also require the involvement of someone trained and skilled to perform the procedure. The principle advantage of comprehensive staging is that the physician and patient are provided with the greatest amount of information. In the contemporary management of endometrial cancer, this information results in less use of radiation, and substitution of vaginal cuff brachytherapy for pelvic RT.

Endometrial cancer is the most common gynecologic malignancy and an understanding of presentation, surgical management, and treatment options is required for any treating practitioners. Surgical therapy is mainstay of endometrial cancer with both pelvic and paraaortic lymphadenectomy recommended with the option to employ minimally invasive surgery in selected patients. Surgical staging largely defines both extent of disease and risk of recurrence. Pelvic radiation is associated with better local control, but no improvement in survival for patients with stage I–II endometrial cancer in randomized trials and complete lymphadenectomy decreases use of postoperative RT.

■ REFERENCES

1. Jemal A, Siegel R, Xu J, Ward E. Cancer statistics, 2010. *CA: Cancer J Clinician.* 2010;60:277–300.

2. Trimble EL, Harlan LC, Clegg LX, et al. Pre-operative imaging, surgery and adjuvant therapy for women diagnosed with cancer of the corpus uteri in community practice in the United States. *Gynecol Oncol.* 2005;96:741–748.

3. Creasman WT, Odicino F, Maisonneuve P, et al. Carcinoma of the corpus uteri. FIGO 26th Annual Report on the Results of Treatment in Gynecological Cancer. *Int J Gynecol Obstet.* 2006;95 (Suppl 1):S105–S143.

4. Heyman J. The so-called Stockholm Method and the results of treatment of uterine cancer at the Radiumhemmet. *Acta Radiol.* 1935;16:129.

5. Arneson AN, Stanbro WW, Nolan JF. The use of multiple sources of radium within the uterus in the treatment of endometrial cancer. *Am J Obstet Gynecol.* 1948;55:64.

6. Asbury RF, Blessing JA, McGuire WP, et al. Aminothiadiazole (NSC 4728) in patients with advanced carcinoma of the endometrium. A phase II study of the Gynecologic Oncology group. *Am J Clin Oncol.* 1990;13:39–41.

7. Nolan J, Arneson A. An instrument for inserting multiple capsules of radium within the uterus in the treatment of corpus cancers. *Am J Roentgenol.* 1943;49:504.

8. Barakat RR, Lev G, Hummer AJ, et al. Twelve-year experience in the management of endometrial cancer: A change in surgical and postoperative radiation approaches. *Gynecol Oncol.* 2007;105:150–156.

9. Dobbie BTC, Waterhouse J. Study of carcinoma of the endometrium. *J Obstet Gynaecol Br Commonw.* 1973;114:106–109.

10. Gray L. Lymph node excision in treatment of gynecologic malignancies. *Am J Surg.* 1964;108:660–663.

11. Lewis GC, Jr., Bundy B. Surgery for endometrial cancer. *Cancer.* 1981;48(2 Suppl):568–574.

12. Naumann RW, Coleman RL. The use of adjuvant radiation therapy in early endometrial cancer by members of the Society of Gynecologic Oncologists in 2005. *Gynecol Oncol.* 2007;105(1):7–12.

13. Creasman WT, Morrow CP, Bundy BN, et al. Surgical pathologic spread patterns of endometrial cancer. A Gynecologic Oncology Group Study. *Cancer.* 1987;60(8 Suppl):2035–2041.

14. Morrow CP, Bundy BN, Kurman RJ, et al. Relationship between surgical-pathological risk factors and outcome in clinical stage I and II carcinoma of the endometrium: A Gynecologic Oncology Group study. *Gynecol Oncol.* 1991;40:55–65.

15. Abeler VM, Kjorstad KE. Endometrial adenocarcinoma in Norway. A study of a total population. *Cancer.* 1991;67(12):3093–3103.

16. Baak JP, Mutter GL, Robboy S, et al. The molecular genetics and morphometry-based endometrial intra-epithelial neoplasia classification system predicts disease progression in endometrial hyperplasia more accurately than the 1994 World Health Organization classification system. *Cancer.* 2005;103(11):2304–2312.

17. Boronow RC, Morrow CP, Creasman WT, et al. Surgical staging in endometrial cancer: Clinical-pathologic findings of a prospective study. *Obstet Gynecol.* 1984;63:825–832.

18. Gal D, Recio FO, Zamurovic D. The new International Federation of Gynecology and Obstetrics surgical staging and survival rates in early endometrial carcinoma. *Cancer.* 1992;69:200–202.

19. Homesley HD, Zaino R. Endometrial cancer: Prognostic factors. *Semin Oncol.* 1994;21:71–78.

20. Kosary CL. FIGO stage, histology, histologic grade, age and race as prognostic factors in determining survival for cancers of the female gynecological system: an analysis of 1973–87 SEER cases of cancers of the endometrium, cervix, ovary, vulva, and vagina. *Sem Surg Oncol.* 1994;10:31–46.

21. Wolfson AH, Sightler SE, Markoe AM, et al. The prognostic significance of surgical staging for carcinoma of the endometrium. *Gynecol Oncol.* 1992;45:142–146.

22. Zaino RJ, Kurman RJ, Diana KL, et al. Pathologic models to predict outcome for women with endometrial adenocarcinoma: The importance of the distinction between surgical stage and clinical stage—a Gynecologic Oncology Group study. *Cancer.* 1996;77:1115–11121.

23. Mariani A, Webb MJ, Keeney GL, et al. Stage IIIC endometrioid corpus cancer includes distinct subgroups. *Gynecol Oncol.* 2002;87:112–117.

24. McMeekin DS, Lashbrook D, Gold M, et al. Analysis of FIGO Stage IIIc endometrial cancer patients. *Gynecol Oncol.* 2001;81:273–278.

25. Chuang L, Burke TW, Tornos C, et al. Staging laparotomy for endometrial carcinoma: Assessment of retroperitoneal lymph nodes. *Gynecol Oncol.* 1995;58:189–193.

26. Mariani A, Dowdy SC, Cliby WA, et al. Efficacy of systematic lymphadenectomy and adjuvant radiotherapy in node-positive endometrial cancer patients. *Gynecol Oncol.* 2006;101:200–208.

27. Onda T, Yoshikawa H, Mizutani K, et al. Treatment of node-positive endometrial cancer with complete node dissection, chemotherapy and radiation therapy. *Br J Cancer.* 1997;75:1836–1841.

28. Havrilesky LJ, Cragun JM, Calingaert B, et al. Resection of lymph node metastases influences survival in stage IIIC endometrial cancer. *Gynecol Oncol.* 2005;99:689–695.

29. Kitchener H. ASTEC—A study in the treatment of endometrial cancer: A randomised trial of lymphadenectomy in the treatment of endometrial cancer [abstract]. *Gynecol Oncol.* 101(1 Suppl 1):S21–22.

30. Randall ME, Filiaci VL, Muss H, et al. Randomized phase III trial of whole-abdominal irradiation versus doxorubicin and cisplatin chemotherapy in advanced endometrial carcinoma: A Gynecologic Oncology Group Study. *J Clin Oncol.* 2006;24:36–44.

31. Takeshima N, Umayahara K, Fujiwara K, et al. Effectiveness of postoperative chemotherapy for para-aortic lymph node metastasis of endometrial cancer. *Gynecol Oncol.* 2006;102(2):214–217.

32. Ben-Shachar I, Pavelka J, Cohn DE, et al. Surgical staging for patients presenting with grade 1 endometrial carcinoma. *Obstet Gynecol.* 2005;105:487–493.

33. Goudge C, Bernhard S, Cloven NG, et al. The impact of complete surgical staging on adjuvant treatment decisions in endometrial cancer. *Gynecol Oncol.* 2004;93: 536–539.

34. Cho H, Kim YT, Kim J-H. Accuracy of preoperative tests in clinical stage I endometrial cancer: The importance of lymphadenectomy. *Acta Obstet Gynecologica Scandinavica.* 2010;89:175–181.

35. Hricak H, Rubinstein LV, Gherman GM, et al. MR imaging evaluation of endometrial carcinoma: Results of an NCI cooperative study. *Radiology.* 1991;179:829–832.

36. Park J-Y, Kim EN, Kim D-Y, et al. Comparison of the validity of magnetic resonance imaging and positron emission tomography/computed tomography in the preoperative evaluation of patients with uterine corpus cancer. *Gynecol Oncol.* 2008;108:486–492.

37. Signorelli M, Guerra L, Buda A, et al. Role of the integrated FDG PET/CT in the surgical management of patients with high risk clinical early stage endometrial cancer: Detection of pelvic nodal metastases. *Gynecol Oncol.* 2009;115:231–235.

38. Girardi F, Petru E, Heydarfadai M, et al. Pelvic lymphadenectomy in the surgical treatment of endometrial cancer. *Gynecol Oncol.* 1993;49:177–180.

39. Tangjitgamol S, Manusirivithaya S, Jesadapatarakul S, et al. Lymph node size in uterine cancer: A revisit. *Int J Gynecol Cancer.* 2006;16:1880–1884.

40. Arango HA, Hoffman MS, Roberts WS, et al. Accuracy of lymph node palpation to determine need for lymphadenectomy in gynecologic malignancies. *Obstet Gynecol.* 2000;95:553–556.

41. Eltabbakh GH. Intraoperative clinical evaluation of lymph nodes in women with gynecologic cancer. *American Journal of Obstetrics & Gynecology,* 2001;184(6):1177–1181.

42. Mariani A, Webb MJ, Keeney GL, et al. Low-risk corpus cancer: Is lymphadenectomy or radiotherapy necessary? *Am J Obstet Gynecol.* 2000;182:1506–1519.

43. Institute NC. Priorities of the Gynecologic Cancer Progress Review Group. 2001.

44. Partridge EE, Shingleton HM, Menck HR. The National Cancer Data Base report on endometrial cancer. *J Surg Oncol.* 1996;61:111–123.

45. Aalders JG, Thomas G. Endometrial cancer—revisiting the importance of pelvic and para aortic lymph nodes. *Gynecol Oncol.* 2007;104:222–231.

46. Creutzberg CL, van Putten WL, Koper PC, et al. Surgery and postoperative radiotherapy versus surgery alone for patients with stage-1 endometrial carcinoma: multicentre randomised trial. PORTEC Study Group. Post Operative Radiation Therapy in Endometrial Carcinoma. *Lancet.* 2000;355:1404–1411.

47. Trimble EL, Kosary C, Park RC. Lymph node sampling and survival in endometrial cancer. *Gynecol Oncol.* 1998;71:340–343.

48. Cosa-Nz-Uk Endometrial Cancer Study Group. Pelvic lymphadenectomy in high risk endometrial cancer. *Int J Gynecol Cancer.* 1996;6:102–107.

49. The ASTEC/EN.5 writing committee. Adjuvant external beam radiotherapy in the treatment of endometrial cancer (MRC ASTEC and NCIC CTG EN.5 randomised trials): Pooled trial results, systematic review, and meta-analysis. *Lancet.* 2009;373:137–146.

50. The writing committee on behalf of the ASTEC study group. Efficacy of systematic pelvic lymphadenectomy in endometrial cancer (MRC ASTEC trial): A randomised study. *Lancet.* 2009;373(9658):125–136.

51. Benedetti Panici P, Basile S, Maneschi F, et al. Systematic pelvic lymphadenectomy vs. no lymphadenectomy in early-stage endometrial carcinoma: Randomized clinical trial. *J Natl Cancer Instit.* 2008;100:1707–1716.

52. Creutzberg CL, van Putten WLJ, Warlam-Rodenhuis CC, et al. Outcome of high-risk stage IC, grade 3, compared with stage I endometrial carcinoma patients: The Postoperative Radiation Therapy in Endometrial Carcinoma Trial. *J Clin Oncol.* 2004;22:1234–1241.

53. Nelson G, Randall M, Sutton G, et al. FIGO stage IIIC endometrial carcinoma with metastases confined to pelvic lymph nodes: Analysis of treatment outcomes, prognostic variables, and failure patterns following adjuvant radiation therapy. *Gynecol Oncol.* 1999;75:211–214.

54. Faught W, Krepart GV, Lotocki R, et al. Should selective paraaortic lymphadenectomy be part of surgical staging for endometrial cancer? *Gynecol Oncol.* 1994;55:51–55.

55. Kim YB, Niloff JM. Endometrial carcinoma: Analysis of recurrence in patients treated with a strategy minimizing lymph node sampling and radiation therapy. *Obstet Gynecol.* 1993;82:175–180.

56. Podratz KC, Mariani A, Webb MJ. Staging and therapeutic value of lymphadenectomy in endometrial cancer. *Gynecol Oncol.* 1998;70:163–164.

57. Goff BA, Kato D, Schmidt RA, et al. Uterine papillary serous carcinoma: Patterns of metastatic spread. *Gynecol Oncol.* 1994;54:264–268.

58. Mariani A, Webb MJ, Galli L, et al. Potential therapeutic role of para-aortic lymphadenectomy in node-positive endometrial cancer. *Gynecol Oncol.* 2000;76:348–356.

59. Flanagan CW, Mannel RS, Walker JL, et al. Incidence and location of para-aortic lymph node metastases in gynecologic malignancies. *J Am Coll Surg.* 1995;181:72–74.

60. McMeekin DS, Lashbrook D, Gold M, et al. Nodal distribution and its significance in FIGO stage IIIc endometrial cancer. *Gynecol Oncol.* 2001;82:375–379.

61. Creasman WT, Zaino RJ, Major FJ, et al. Early invasive carcinoma of the cervix (3 to 5 mm invasion): Risk factors and prognosis. A Gynecologic Oncology Group study. *Am J Obstet Gynecol.* 1998;178(1 Pt 1):62–65.

62. Leblanc E, Querleu D, Narducci F, et al. Surgical staging of early invasive epithelial ovarian tumors. *Sem Surg Oncol.* 2000;19:36–41.

63. Hirahatake K, Hareyama H, Sakuragi N, et al. A clinical and pathologic study on para-aortic lymph node metastasis in endometrial carcinoma. *J Surg Oncol.* 1997;65:82–87.

64. Kilgore LC, Partridge EE, Alvarez RD, et al. Adenocarcinoma of the endometrium: Survival comparisons of patients with and without pelvic node sampling. *Gynecol Oncol.* 1995;56:29–33.

65. Cragun JM, Havrilesky LJ, Calingaert B, et al. Retrospective analysis of selective lymphadenectomy in apparent early-stage endometrial cancer. *J Clin Oncol.* 2005;23:3668–3675.

66. Keys HM, Roberts JA, Brunetto VL, et al. A phase III trial of surgery with or without adjunctive external pelvic radiation therapy in intermediate risk endometrial adenocarcinoma: A Gynecologic Oncology Group study. *Gynecol Oncol.* 2004;92:744–751.

67. Fanning J, Nanavati PJ, Hilgers RD. Surgical staging and high dose rate brachytherapy for endometrial cancer: Limiting external radiotherapy to node-positive tumors. *Obstet Gynecol.* 1996;87:1041–1044.

68. Mohan DS, Samuels MA, Selim MA, et al. Long-term outcomes of therapeutic pelvic lymphadenectomy for stage I endometrial adenocarcinoma. *Gynecol Oncol.* 1998;70:165–171.

69. Orr JW, Jr., Holimon JL, Orr PF. Stage I corpus cancer: Is teletherapy necessary? *Am J Obstet Gynecol.* 1997;176:777–788.

70. Singh M, Zaino RJ, Filiaci VJ, et al. Relationship of estrogen and progesterone receptors to clinical outcome in metastatic endometrial carcinoma: A Gynecologic Oncology Group Study. *Gynecol Oncol.* 2007;106:325–333.

71. Walker JL, Piedmonte MR, Spirtos NM, et al. Laparoscopy compared with laparotomy for comprehensive surgical staging of uterine cancer: Gynecologic Oncology Group Study LAP2. *J Clin Oncol.* 2009;27:5331–5336.

72. Gemignani ML, Curtin JP, Zelmanovich J, et al. Laparoscopic-assisted vaginal hysterectomy for endometrial cancer: Clinical outcomes and hospital charges. *Gynecol Oncol.* 1999;73:5–11.

73. Spirtos NM, Schlaerth JB, Gross GM, et al. Cost and quality-of-life analyses of surgery for early endometrial cancer: Laparotomy versus laparoscopy. *Am J Obstet Gynecol.* 1996;174:1795–1799.

74. Fowler JM, Carter JR, Carlson JW, et al. Lymph node yield from laparoscopic lymphadenectomy in cervical cancer: A comparative study. *Gynecol Oncol.* 1993;51:187–192.

75. Bell MC, Torgerson J, Seshadri-Kreaden U, et al. Comparison of outcomes and cost for endometrial cancer staging via traditional laparotomy, standard laparoscopy and robotic techniques. *Gynecol Oncol.* 2008;111:407–411.

76. Boggess JF, Gehrig PA, Cantrell L, et al. A comparative study of 3 surgical methods for hysterectomy with staging for endometrial cancer: Robotic assistance, laparoscopy, laparotomy. *Am J Obstet Gynecol.* 2008;199: 360–364.

77. Reza M, Maeso S, Blasco JA, et al. Meta-analysis of observational studies on the safety and effectiveness of robotic gynaecological surgery. *Br J Surg.* 2010;97:1772–1783.

78. Seamon LG, Cohn DE, Henretta MS, et al. Minimally invasive comprehensive surgical staging for endometrial cancer: Robotics or laparoscopy? *Gynecol Oncol.* 2009;113:36–41.

79. Veljovich DS, Paley PJ, Drescher CW, et al. Robotic surgery in gynecologic oncology: program initiation and outcomes after the first year with comparison with laparotomy for endometrial cancer staging. *Am J Obstet Gynecol.* 2008;198:679–684.

80. Khoury Collado F, Abu-Rustum NR. Lymphatic mapping in endometrial cancer: A literaturere view of current techniques and results. *Int J Gynecol Cancer.* 2008;18:1163–1168.

81. Robison K, Holman LL, Moore RG. Update on sentinel lymph node evaluation in gynecologic malignancies. *Curr Opin Obstet Gynecol.* 2011;23:8–12.

82. Ballester M, Dubernard G, Lecuru F, et al. Detection rate and diagnostic accuracy of sentinel-node biopsy in early stage endometrial cancer: A prospective multicentre study (SENTI-ENDO). *Lancet Oncol.* 2011;12:469–476.

83. Abu-Rustum NR, Alektiar K, Iasonos A, et al. The incidence of symptomatic lower-extremity lymphedema following treatment of uterine corpus malignancies: A 12-year experience at Memorial Sloan-Kettering Cancer Center. *Gynecol Oncol.* 2006;103:714–718.

84. Homesley HD, Kadar N, Barrett RJ, et al. Selective pelvic and periaortic lymphadenectomy does not increase morbidity in surgical staging of endometrial carcinoma. *Am J Obstet Gynecol.* 1992;167:1225–1230.

85. Lewandowski G, Torrisi J, Potkul RK, et al. Hysterectomy with extended surgical staging and radiotherapy versus hysterectomy alone and radiotherapy in stage I endometrial cancer: A comparison of complication rates. *Gynecol Oncol.* 1990;36:401–404.

86. Schorge JO, Molpus KL, Goodman A, et al. The effect of postsurgical therapy on stage III endometrial carcinoma. *Gynecol Oncol.* 1996;63:34–39.

87. Otsuka I, Kubota T, Aso T. Lymphadenectomy and adjuvant therapy in endometrial carcinoma: Role of adjuvant chemotherapy. *Br J Cancer.* 2002;87:377–380.

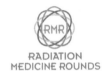

Robotic Surgery in Gynecologic Cancer

Marilyn Huang and Pedro Ramirez*

*Department of Gynecologic Oncology & Reproductive Medicine,
MD Anderson Cancer Center, Houston, TX*

■ ABSTRACT

In the last several decades, operative laparoscopy has become an accepted alternative approach to traditional laparotomy. Robotic systems enhance the surgeon's ability to manipulate instruments, scale movements so that large
movements of the control grips are transformed into micromotions within the patient, and restore hand–eye coordination. This modality has significantly impacted minimally invasive surgery for patients with gynecologic malignancies, and this chapter provides an overview of the current utilization.

Keywords: robotic surgery, gynecologic oncology

■ INTRODUCTION

Minimally invasive surgery has become widely
accepted as a standard modality in the management
of patients with most gynecologic malignancies. The
advantages of laparoscopic surgery quickly gained
popularity among surgeons and patients due to the
smaller incisions, lower risk of infection, less blood
loss, and shorter hospital stays. While laparoscopy
has afforded many additional advantages including
faster return of bowel function, faster overall recovery time, fewer complications, and better results,
there are distinct disadvantages. Surgeons are limited
to a two-dimensional (2D) view of the surgical field,
rigid instruments without articulation or rotation,

fatigue due to poor ergonomics, and potentially a
long learning curve (1,2).

More recently, robotic surgery has come to the
forefront of surgical innovation. The DaVinci robotic
system (Intuitive Surgical Inc., Sunnyvale, CA) was
approved by the Food and Drug Administration
(FDA) for use in gynecologic surgery in 2005. The
robotic system provides a range of advantages over
laparoscopy, such as seven degrees of motion, 3D
views, tremor filtration, improved dexterity, and surgeon comfort. The robotic system consists of three
components: (a) a surgeon console with an integrated three-dimensional (3D) display (Figure 1),
(b) a vision system equipped with high-definition 3D
endoscope and a monitor to view the operating field
for the entire operating room (OR) team (Figure 2),
and (c) a patient-side cart with either three or four
robotic arms (Figure 3). This system allows the primary surgeon to view the surgical field on a 3D screen
and manipulate the robotic arms using hand-held

---

*Corresponding author, Department of Gynecologic
Oncology & Reproductive Medicine, MD Anderson Cancer
Center, 1155 Pressler Dr, Unit 1362, Houston, TX 77230
    E-mail address: peramire@mdanderson.org

Radiation Medicine Rounds 2:3 (2011) 439–448.
DOI: 10.5003/2151–4208.2.3.439

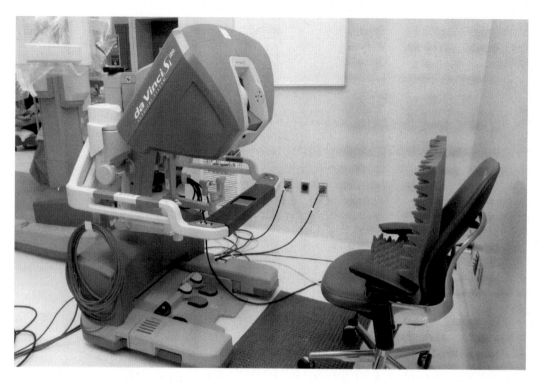

FIGURE 1 Surgeon console.

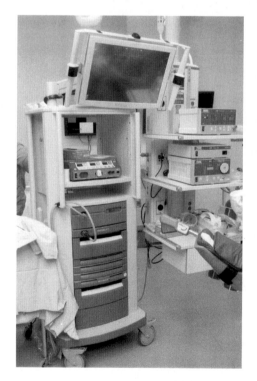

FIGURE 2 Vision system including 3-D viewing screen.

controls within the console (Figure 1) (3). The latest version of the robotic system was introduced in 2009, the DaVinci Si system, featuring a dual console to support training and collaboration during minimally invasive surgery (Figure 4). The Si model also incorporates an enhanced 3D high-definition resolution that enhances visualization, providing the surgeon with even greater surgical precision (4). Overall, robotic systems enhance the surgeon's ability to manipulate instruments, scale movements so that large movements of the control grips are transformed into micromotions within the patient, and restore hand–eye coordination.

The volume of data being generated on robotic surgery is multiplying and early data are promising. Several studies have compared the outcomes in women undergoing surgical management of gynecologic malignancies by laparotomy, laparoscopy, or robotic-assisted surgery.

■ ADOPTION OF ROBOTIC SURGERY

The number of robotic-assisted procedures performed worldwide has nearly tripled since 2007, from

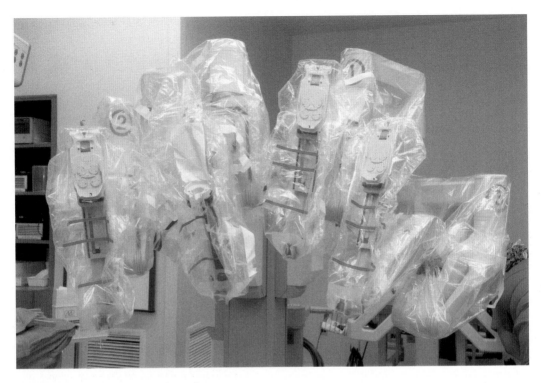

FIGURE 3 Patient-side cart including robotic arms.

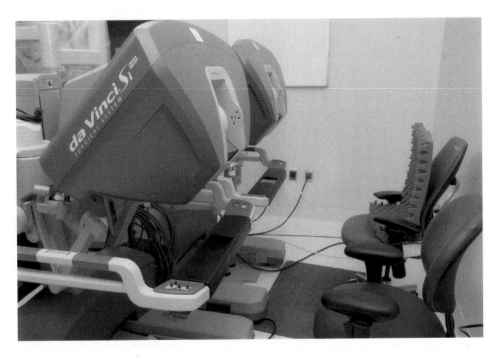

FIGURE 4 Dual surgeon console.

80,000 to 205,000. From 2007 to 2009, the number of robotic systems installed in United States hospitals expanded from 800 to approximately 1400, an increase of about 75% (5). Over 1200 gynecologic surgeons in 2010 alone were trained to use the robotic system (6). In the past 3 years, there have been over 200 articles dedicated to robotics in gynecologic surgery. Thus, the introduction of robotic surgery has markedly transformed practice patterns within the gynecologic oncology community.

■ TRAINING

In robotic surgery, surgeons must first become proficient in port placement (Figure 5a and 5b), set-up, and docking of the robot and then become competent in performing individual procedures. Minimally invasive surgery has primarily been assessed through metrics such as total operative time, estimated blood loss, rate of intraoperative complications, and rate of conversion to laparotomy. However, these parameters may not accurately gauge a surgeon's level of proficiency. For example, as a surgeon becomes more familiar with the robotic system, he/she may begin to perform more technically difficult cases, schedule more challenging patients, or integrate teaching of residents and/or fellows.

In an effort to provide an objective analysis of surgical performance on robot-assisted procedures for endometrial cancer during the learning phase, Holloway et al. examined a cohort of 100 patients, comparing the first 10 cases with the last 10 cases. The authors found that the total lymph node counts increased mostly due to an increased number of paraaortic lymph nodes, and there was a decrease in operative time. There were more grade 3 tumors treated in the last 50 cases (7). These results suggest that as the surgeon gains experience using the robotic system, the operative time decreases and more paraaortic lymph nodes are obtained. Seamon et al. examined the learning curve among endometrial cancer patients that were operated on by a robotic-assisted procedure and determined that in their group, proficiency for robotic hysterectomy with pelvic and paraaortic lymphadenectomy was achieved after 20 cases (8).

Training surgeons in robotic surgery can occur through a variety of modalities. For example, surgeons may acquire knowledge through didactics, online tools, dry laboratory training, and animal laboratory training. Residents and fellows frequently begin their learning process as the patient-side assistant in the OR then progressing to the robotic console. The launch of the robotic surgery program has herald a dramatic shift in case load for fellow training in minimally invasive surgery.

A recent questionnaire survey of gynecologic oncology fellows and fellowship directors demonstrated that robotic surgery was being utilized in the majority of responding programs with an overall favorable view of robotic surgery. Respondents indicated that most were performing between five and eight robotic cases per month for a wide range of indications. Moreover, an overwhelming majority of fellows (94%) planned on performing robotic surgery in their practice (9). Though the survey may not have represented the overall group of practicing gynecologic oncologist as only 30% responded to the survey, it highlights a crucial new component of fellowship education.

Hoekstra et al. described the impact of a new robotic surgery program on the surgical training of gynecologic oncology fellows over a 12-month period at a single institution for the surgical management of endometrial and cervical cancer. The proportion of minimally invasive surgery increased dramatically from 3.3% to 43.5% and fellow participation in robotic procedures increased from 45% at 3 months to 92% by 12 months. Furthermore, the specific role of the fellow transitioned from bedside assistant to console operator within 3 months. Perhaps the most striking aspect of robotic surgery is the relative independence of the trainee when sitting at the console as compared with laparoscopic or open techniques. The authors concluded that while robotic surgery broadens the gynecologic oncologists' surgical capabilities, it may put significant challenges on the training of fellows equally in laparotomy, laparoscopy, and robotic techniques (10).

In general, tools have been developed to enrich training on the robot system. For example, a touchscreen robotic illustrator allows experienced surgeons to add visual cues to the image seen by the trainee inside the console and thereby enhancing trainer–trainee communication and interactions. The ProMis simulator (Haptica, Dublin, Ireland) is a modular virtual reality simulator that was initially constructed for laparoscopic training but has now began testing for robotic surgery training. A recent study provides evidence that ProMis may differentiate between experienced and novice robotic surgeons

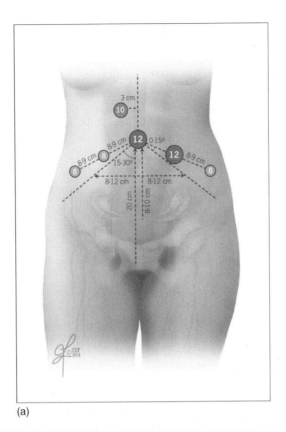

(a)

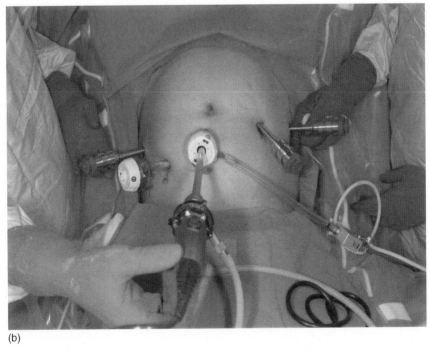

(b)

FIGURE 5 (a) Port placement considerations; (b) port placement example.

when using training models. Smoothness, as measured by number of movements required to complete a task, was the most objective parameter distinguishing between expert and novice surgeons (11). Robotic simulators are currently available for practice in multiple tasks and allow an objective measurement of performance. Furthermore, the recent introduction of the dual surgeon console permits a master-apprentice teaching design more similar to that experienced in laparoscopy or laparotomy.

■ CLINICAL IMPACT: ENDOMETRIUM

The most common use of the robotic system in gynecologic oncology is in the surgical management of endometrial cancer. In a retrospective review of endometrial cancer patients undergoing surgical staging, Boggess et al. found the robotic-assisted approach to be feasible. The authors found that the highest number of lymph nodes, least amount of blood loss, and shortest hospital stay were seen in the robotic group compared with both laparotomy and laparoscopy (12).

In the largest series to date, Gaia et al. conducted a systematic review that included eight comparative studies examining a total of 1,591 patients. Of these, 589 cases were robotic, 396 laparoscopic, and 606 laparotomies. The authors found that estimated blood loss was lower for robotic hysterectomy than for laparoscopy ($p = .001$) or laparotomy ($p < .005$). Length of stay was shorter for both robotic and laparoscopic cases compared with laparotomy ($p < .01$). The operative time for robotic hysterectomy was similar to laparoscopic cases, but significantly greater than laparotomy ($p < .005$). The conversion rate to laparotomy was slightly higher for laparoscopic hysterectomies than for robotic procedures, although this was not statistically significant ($p = .06$). Complications such as vascular, bowel, and bladder injuries; cuff dehiscence; and thromboembolic complications were similar among the three groups. Of note, patients undergoing robotic hysterectomy had the lowest frequency of blood transfusion requirement (1.7%) when compared with laparoscopic (2.6%) or laparotomy (5.0%). The authors thus concluded that clinical outcomes for robotic and laparoscopic hysterectomy appear comparable. However, both minimally invasive approaches required longer operative times when compared with laparotomy (13).

A cohort comparison study of outcomes between robotic and laparoscopic hysterectomy with lymphadenectomy in patients with endometrial cancer revealed that robotic surgery was accomplished in heavier patients with fewer conversions to laparotomy (14). There were 181 patients included (105 robotic and 75 laparoscopic). Patients that underwent robotic surgery had a significantly higher body mass index (BMI), but had less blood loss, lower transfusion rates, lower laparotomy conversion rates, and shorter hospital stays compared with the laparoscopic cohort. Additionally, robotic hysterectomy and lymphadenectomy were performed in a shorter time than when the surgery was performed by laparoscopy (14).

These recent studies have shown that in obese women with endometrial cancer, robotic surgery offers advantages over laparoscopy. In particular, benefits include less blood loss, less transfusion requirements, less frequent rate of conversion to laparotomy, less operative time, and shorter hospital stay (15,16). These studies, however, are retrospective and thus subject to potential selection biases. On the basis of the available data, the predominating consensus in the literature suggests that robotic surgery may be equivalent to laparoscopy. However, since obesity is a significant risk factor for endometrial cancer, and as the prevalence of obesity increases, future studies to ascertain which surgical techniques would be most appropriate to manage these patients are vital.

■ CLINICAL IMPACT: CERVIX

Cervical cancer, the second most common malignancy in women worldwide, is generally treated by an open radical hysterectomy with pelvic lymph node dissection. This procedure is one of the more intricate surgical procedures performed by gynecologic oncologists due to the degree of dissection required. Sert and Abeler described the first robotic-assisted radical hysterectomy and pelvic lymphadenectomy in a patient with early-stage cervical cancer. The authors showed that robotic radical hysterectomy with pelvic lymph node dissection was feasible (17). The authors subsequently published the first comparative study in 15 patients investigating robotic-assisted laparoscopic hysterectomy and pelvic lymphadenectomy with early-stage cervical cancer compared with those undergoing laparoscopy. This study demonstrated that robotic surgery was comparable with the laparoscopic approach as evidenced by less blood loss and shorter hospital stay (18). Subsequently, Boggess et al.

performed a case-control cohort study comparing 51 patients that underwent robotic-assisted radical hysterectomy and 49 patients who underwent laparotomy for early-stage cervical cancer. The authors also found that robotic radical hysterectomy with pelvic node dissection was feasible and may be preferable to open radical hysterectomy (19).

Magrina et al. compared 27 patients who underwent robotic radical hysterectomy for either cervical or endometrial cancer to matched groups treated by laparoscopy and laparotomy. The authors reported similar operating times in the robotic and laparotomy groups, both of which were significantly shorter compared with the laparoscopy group. However, the laparoscopy and robotic groups had significantly less blood loss and length of hospital stay. Overall, there was no significant difference in complication rates among the three groups. The authors concluded that laparoscopy and robotics were preferable to laparotomy for patients requiring radical hysterectomy with some advantages favoring robotic surgery (16). In a similar study by Estape and colleagues, comparing cervical cancer treatment in three groups: robotic-assisted, laparoscopy, and laparotomy. The authors corroborated pervious work demonstrating similar operative time, estimated blood loss, and mean hospital stay of robotic-assisted surgery to be similar to that of laparoscopy. However, in their study, the incidence of postoperative complications was less in the robotic cohort compared with laparoscopy and laparotomy (20). While these early studies are promising, more research is required to evaluate long-term survival and cancer control in this population.

Thus, a large multi-institutional international phase III randomized control trial comparing laparoscopy or robotic radical hysterectomy compared with abdominal hysterectomy for early-stage cervical cancer is in progress. This biphasic study was designed to test the feasibility of recruitment and equivalence in regard to disease-free survival. Patients with documented invasive squamous cell or adenocarcinoma with stage IA1 with lymph-vascular space invasion, IA2, or IB1 are currently being randomized. The primary end-point of this prospective randomized trial is recurrence-free survival (21).

Another procedure that is being performed with increasing frequency in patients with early-stage cervical cancer is the radical trachelectomy. This procedure was initially described by Dargent et al. in 1994 (22). Radical trachelectomy is performed in young women diagnosed with cervical cancer who are interested in future fertility by removing the cervix and parametrial tissue and anastomosing the uterus to the upper vagina. A number of publications have already documented the feasibility of robotic radical trachelectomy. In a case series, four patients underwent robotic radical trachelectomy with bilateral pelvic lymphadenectomy. There were no conversions to laparotomy or intraoperative complications. One patient experienced transient lower extremity sensory neuropathy that spontaneously resolved after about 20 days. None of the patients received adjuvant therapy. The median follow-up time was 105 days, and at the last follow-up, there were no recurrences (23). In another case series, six patients had a robotic radical trachelectomy with bilateral pelvic lymphadenectomy. There were two postoperative complications. One patient had a small bowel hernia through a lateral 8-mm port on day 3 requiring an incision over the port site to release the herniated bowel and to repair the fascial defect. The other patient presented on postoperative day 4 with an anterior abdominal wall ecchymosis consistent with inferior epigastric vessel hemorrhage, which resolved without intervention but a blood transfusion was required. Follow-up ranged from 9 to 13 months with no recurrences or pregnancies at the time of publication (24). These early results have demonstrated that the procedure is associated with minimal blood loss, short length of hospital stays, low rates of intraoperative and postoperative complications with adequate surgical specimens (23,24). Early studies demonstrate feasibility; however, larger studies with long-term oncologic and obstetric outcomes are needed.

■ CLINICAL IMPACT: OVARY

Only a few cases reporting the use of robotic surgery for the management of ovarian cancer are available. Currently, early-stage disease may be more amenable to a robotic approach than advanced disease. Robotic surgery may not be well suited in women with advanced ovarian cancer due to the limited access to the upper abdomen.

In a retrospective case-control analysis, Magrina et al. compared perioperative outcomes and survival in patients undergoing primary surgical treatment for epithelial ovarian cancer by either a robotic, laparoscopic, or laparotomy approach. There were 25 patients that had primary surgical treatment with the robotic approach compared with 27 patients treated by laparoscopy and 119 patients treated by laparotomy. Patients in each surgical group were then further classified into type I, II, or III debulking cohorts according to the extent of surgical debulking performed based on the type and number of major procedures. Type I debulking consisted of hysterectomy, adnexectomy, omentectomy, pelvic and paraaortic lymphadenectomy, appendectomy, and removal of metastatic peritoneal disease if present. Type II debulking was type I plus one other major procedure and type III debulking was type I plus two or more major procedures. Major procedures were defined as any type of intestinal resection, full thickness diaphragm resection, resection of liver disease, and splenectomy.

Patients with early-stage disease undergoing type I debulking demonstrated improved perioperative outcomes when robotic or laparoscopy was utilized (less blood loss and shorter hospital stay) compared with laparotomy. Operating times and complications were similar across all three groups. For type II debulking patients, the robotic and laparoscopy groups both had less blood loss, fewer complications, and shorter hospital stays compared with the laparotomy group. Only robotic and laparotomy approaches were used for the type III debulking procedures. In the type III group, patients that underwent robotic surgery had less blood loss and less intraoperative complications but longer operating time and more postoperative complications. Lengths of hospital stay for type III debulked patients were similar regardless of approach. Thus, the authors concluded that robotic and laparoscopic approaches may be promising for the surgical management of ovarian cancer but for those requiring extensive debulking, laparotomy remains preferable (25).

■ COST

One of the biggest concerns regarding the adoption of robotic technology is the high cost. Robotic surgical systems currently have high fixed costs, ranging from $1 million to $2.5 million for each unit. The current list price of a DaVinci Si is approximately $1.75 million (5). The systems require costly maintenance and require training for team members. The annual maintenance fees are approximately $140,000 and include quarterly maintenance checks along with replacement of parts that malfunction or break. Additionally, Intuitive Surgical is the sole manufacturer of robotic surgical devices keeping prices fixed.

The impact of robotic technology on the healthcare system remains to be determined (5). Ideally, when comparing costs between robotic-assisted surgery to other approaches of surgery, direct and indirect costs should both be factored. The fixed cost of a robotic system is usually amortized over its expected lifespan, differing from the fixed costs of laparoscopy and open procedures. Other costs to be considered between robotic, laparoscopy, and open surgery are costs of OR supplies and equipment, operating and recovery room time, physician fees, and all hospitals fees including room and board. Additionally, costs due to complications and loss of productivity while recovering should be incorporated.

In a decision-modeling study, Barnett et al., compared the costs associated with robotic, laparoscopic, and laparotomies for the treatment of endometrial cancer. The authors used three models: (a) a societal perspective model that included inpatient hospital costs, robotic expenses, lost wages, and caregiver costs; (b) a hospital perspective plus robot costs model that is the societal perspective model minus the lost wages and caregiver costs; and (c) a hospital perspective without robot costs model, which is similar to the hospital perspective plus robot costs except initial cost of the robot was excluded. The authors found that the societal perspective model predicted laparoscopy to be the least expensive followed by robotic and open laparotomy. The hospital perspective plus robot costs model yielded similar results unless the hospital stay for the laparotomy was less than 2.9 days. The hospital perspective without robot costs model also favored laparoscopy as least expensive unless the cost of robotic disposable equipment was kept to less than $1,496 per case. The authors thus concluded that laparoscopic surgery for endometrial cancer treatment was the least-expensive approach (26). Interestingly, the most important factor in this study driving the relative costs in each model was the time to return to full activity and the cost of disposable equipment.

In general, minimally invasive surgery is less costly than open procedures when associated costs such as duration of hospital stay and recovery time are included. Within minimally invasive surgery, robot-assisted procedures are normally more expensive than laparoscopic procedures secondary to the costs and employment of more disposable material.

OR time is also a key aspect to minimizing the cost of robotic surgery; as surgeons and staff become more proficient, operating time may be significantly less than laparoscopy. A prospective matched case-control study examined perioperative outcomes and costs of robotic surgery compared with laparoscopic hysterectomies for benign indications. The authors found that robotic hysterectomy was feasible and had comparable outcomes to laparoscopy. Total costs for robotic surgery were higher than for laparoscopy and was mostly attributed to material costs (26). However, studies analyzing cost-effectiveness are small and few, making valid evaluation difficult.

FUTURE

As the use of robotic surgery in the treatment of gynecologic cancers continues to expand, it is important to examine both credentialing and the medical-legal aspects of using the robot. Currently, there is no standard for credentialing among robotic surgeons. The American College of Surgeons has proposed general guidelines for introducing new technology into surgical practice. The guidelines include: (a) assessing a surgeon's eligibility to use the new technology on the basis of previous training and experience, (b) require education to ensure adequate understanding of the new technology, and (c) ensure an environment appropriate for the use of the new technology. As robotic surgery develops, high-quality cost–benefit assessments regarding the use of robotic surgery are needed. Previously published studies report primarily on perioperative and short-term postoperative results; thus, leaving the long-term data piece of the puzzle uncharted.

In conclusion, current evidence supports equivalence of robotic surgery and laparoscopy in perioperative outcomes and a distinct advantage over open surgery in the management of patients with gynecologic cancer. The cost of robotic technology remains a barrier to widespread acceptance, but overall cost may decrease with increasing utilization. More research is required to establish benefits in clinical outcomes. Fellowship programs should include standardized training in both robotic surgery and traditional laparoscopic surgery. We must strive to implement clear guidelines for training to assure patient safety and proper credentialing in all institutions.

REFERENCES

1. Ramirez P, Soliman P, Schmeler K, et al. Laparoscopic and robotic techniques for radical hysterectomy in patients in early-stage cervical cancer. *Gynecol Oncol.* 2008;110:S21–S24.
2. Cho JE, Nezhat FR. Robotics and gynecologic oncology: Review of the literature. *J Minim Invasive Gynecol.* 2009;16:669–681.
3. http://www.intuitivesurgical.com/products/davinci_surgical_system (accessed, 6/1/11).
4. Gastrich MD, Barone M, Bachmann G, et al. Robotic surgery: Review of the latest advances, risks, and outcomes. *J Robotic Surg.* 2011;5:79–97.
5. Cadiere GB, Himpens J, Germay O, et al. Feasibility of robotic laparoscopic surgery: 146 cases. *World J Surg.* 2001;25:1467–1477.
6. Barbash GI, Glied SA. New technology and health care costs—The case of robot-assisted surgery. *N Engl J Med.* 2010;363;701–704.
7. Holloway RW, Ahmad S, DeNardis SA, et al. Robotic-assisted laparoscopic hysterectomy and lymphadenectomy for endometrial cancer: Analysis of surgical performance. *Gynecol Oncol.* 2009;115:447–452.
8. Seamon LG, Fowler JM, Richardson DL, et al. A detailed analysis of the learning curve: robotic hysterectomy and pelvic-aortic lymphadenectomy for endometrial cancer. *Gynecol Oncol.* 2009;114:162–167.
9. Sfakianos GP, Frederick PJ, Kendrick JE, et al. Robotic surgery in gynecologic oncology fellowship programs in the USA: A survey of fellows and fellowship directors. *Int J Med Robot.* 2010;6:405–412.
10. Hoekstra AV, Morgan JM, Lurain JR. Robotic surgery in gynecologic oncology: Impact on fellowship training. *Gynecol Oncol.* 2009;114:168–172.
11. Jonsson MN, Mahmood M, Askerud T, et al. ProMIS can serve as a da Vinci Simulator—A construct validity study. *J Endourol.* 2011;25:345–350.
12. Boggess JF, Gehrig PA, Cantrell L, et al. A comparative study of 3 surgical methods for hysterectomy with staging for endometrial cancer: Robotic assistance, laparoscopy, laparotomy. *Am J Obstet Gynecol.* 2008;199:360–366.
13. Gaia G, Holloway RW, Santoro L, et al. Robotic-assisted hysterectomy for endometrial cancer compared with traditional laparoscopic and laparotomy approaches: A systematic review. *Obstet Gynecol.* 2010;116:1422–1431.
14. Seamon LG, Cohn DE, Henretta MS, et al. Minimally invasive comprehensive surgical staging for endometrial cancer: Robotics or laparoscopy? *Gynecol Oncol.* 2009;113:36–41.
15. Gehrig PA, Cantrell LA, Shafer A, et al. What is the optimal minimally invasive surgical procedure for endometrial cancer staging in the obese and morbidly obese woman? *Gynecol Oncol.* 2008;111:41–45.

16. Magrina JF, Kho RM, Weaver AL, et al. Robotic radical hysterectomy: Comparison with laparoscopy and laparotomy. *Gynecol Oncol.* 2008;109:86–91.

17. Sert BM, Abeler VM. Robotic-assisted laparoscopic radical hysterectomy (Piver type III) with pelvic node dissection-case report. *Eur J Gynaecol Oncol.* 2006;27:531–533.

18. Sert B, Abeler V. Robotic radical hysterectomy in early-stage cervical carcinoma patients, comparing results with total laparoscopic radical hysterectomy cases. The future is now? *Int J Med Robot.* 2007;3:224–228.

19. Boggess JF, Gehrig PA, Cantrell L, et al. A case-control study of robot-assisted type III radical hysterectomy with pelvic lymph node dissection compared with open radical hysterectomy. *Am J Obstet Gynecol.* 2008;199:357–363.

20. Estape R, Lambrou N, Diaz R, et al. A case matched analysis of robotic radical hysterectomy with lymphadenectomy compared with laparoscopy and laparotomy. *Gynecol Oncol.* 2009;113:357–361.

21. Obermair A, Gebski V, Frumovitz M, et al. A phase III randomized clinical trial comparing laparoscopic or robotic radical hysterectomy with abdominal radical hysterectomy in patients with early stage cervical cancer. *J Minim Invasive Gynecol.* 2008;15:584–588.

22. Dargent D, Brun J, Roy M, Remy I. Pregnancies following radical trachelectomy for invasive cervical cancer. *Gynecol Oncol.* 1994;52:105 [Abstract].

23. Ramirez PT, Schmeler KM, Malpica A, et al. Safety and feasibility of robotic radical trachelectomy in patients with early-stage cervical cancer. *Gynecol Oncol.* 2010;116:512–515.

24. Burnett AF, Stone PJ, Duckworth LA, et al. Robotic radical trachelectomy for preservation of fertility in early cervical cancer: case series and description of technique. *J Minim Invasive Gynecol.* 2009;16:569–572.

25. Magrina JF, Zanagnolo V, Noble BN, et al. Robotic approach for ovarian cancer: Perioperative and survival results and comparison with laparoscopy and laparotomy. *Gynecol Oncol.* 2010;121:100–105.

26. Barnett JC, Judd JP, Wu JM, et al. Cost comparison among robotic, laparoscopic, and open hysterectomy for endometrial cancer. *Obstet Gynecol.* 2010;116: 685–693.

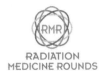

RADIATION
MEDICINE ROUNDS

Magnetic Resonance Imaging for Assessing Tumor Response in Cervical Cancer

Nina A. Mayr,[1]* Zhibin Huang,[2] Simon S. Lo,[3] and William T. C. Yuh[4]

[1]*Department of Radiation Oncology, Ohio State University, Columbus, OH;*
[2]*Department of Radiation Oncology, East Carolina University, Greenville, NC;*
[3]*Department of Radiation Oncology, Case Western Reserve University,*
Cleveland, OH; and [4]*Department of Radiology, Ohio State University, Columbus, OH*

■ ABSTRACT

This chapter will review magnetic resonance imaging (MRI)-based morphologic tumor volume imaging in cervical cancer and its regression for treatment response assessment and prediction of patient outcome. The role of clinical functional MRI, including the dynamic contrast enhanced (DCE) MRI and diffusion weighted imaging (DWI), in the assessment of the functional/biological properties of the tumor will be discussed. With the new ability to quantify early subtle morphologic and functional/biological changes, prediction of ultimate treatment outcomes, local recurrence and survival, to the ongoing therapy can be made as early as 2 to 5 weeks into the chemoradiotherapy course. Furthermore, MRI-based early response and predictive parameters can be significantly enhanced by synergizing information from both morphologic and functional/biological MRI parameters, and further increased by augmenting these with readily available established clinical prognostic factors, including tumor stage and lymph node status.

Keywords: magnetic resonance imaging, functional, uterine cervical neoplasms, radiotherapy

■ INTRODUCTION

Response assessment of chemoradiotherapy in cervical cancer has relied on the measurement of tumor size and tumor regression, largely derived from physical examination. Tumor palpation has limited accuracy, which is further compromised by fibrosis and anatomical distortion induced by the cytotoxic treatment. More recently cross-sectional imaging has supplemented clinical examination-based assessments, using imaging-based tumor diameters (1,2), without considering tumor irregularity. However, determination of treatment failure with these methods can frequently not be made until many months or even years after the completion of treatment. At that time, salvage therapy options are usually limited, mostly ineffective, and the vast majority of patients die after failed therapy

*Corresponding author, Department of Radiation Oncology, Ohio State University, Arthur G. James Cancer Hospital and Solove Research Institute, 300 W 10th Ave, Rm. 088B, Columbus, OH 43210

E-mail address: Nina.Mayr@osumc.edu
Conflict of Interest: This research is supported by NIH (contract grant number: RO1 CA 71906)

Radiation Medicine Rounds 2:3 (2011) 449–462.
DOI: 10.5003/2151–4208.2.3.449

(3). Despite the increasing availability of intensified therapy options (dose intensification of radiation and brachytherapy, cytotoxic radiosensitizing, or targeted agents) (4–7), salvage therapies cannot be implemented in a timely and targeted fashion without an early predictor of treatment failure risk. Therefore the prediction of ultimate treatment failure at the *earliest possible time* is key to improving treatment outcome. Such early personalized information provides a therapeutic window for targeted adaptive therapy.

To achieve a reliable response assessment and outcome prediction, the ability to detect subtle morphologic and functional/biological tumor changes during an ongoing treatment is essential, so that outcome prediction can be made during the *early* therapy phase.

With the improvement of three-dimensional (3D) spatial resolution in clinical cross-sectional imaging, more precise measurement of tumor volume and its regression can now be achieved. In addition, more readily available novel advanced functional imaging techniques can provide noninvasive physiological/biological assessment and detect subtle early functional tumor changes in response to therapy, that greatly improve response assessment and the *early* prediction of therapy outcome.

■ ANATOMICAL TUMOR VOLUME ASSESSMENT BY MRI

Computed tomography (CT) cannot differentiate the cervical tumor from the normal cervix and uterus (8–10) and thus is not well-suited for tumor volume measurement. MRI provides multi-planar ability, superb anatomical detail and tissue contrast between the tumor, uterus, and surrounding normal structures, and therefore is an ideal imaging modality to delineate cervical tumors and derive tumor volume measurements (8–14). In MRI–histologic correlation studies, a 98% correlation was reported between 3D MRI-based tumor volume and digitized histologic tumor volume from giant tissue sections (11,12). This high-precision 3D delineation makes MRI the gold standard for tumor volume measurement in cervical cancer.

Tumor Volume, Volume Response Assessment, and Early Outcome Prediction

The overall importance of tumor size on local control and survival following treatment in cervical cancer is well-documented (15–18). Both local control and survival can profoundly change within the same stage category based on tumor size (15,18). Several groups have studied anatomic tumor volume regression during radiation therapy (RT) in cervical cancer (19–23). Despite variable tumor measurement techniques, tumor regression has been shown to correlate with final tumor response and ultimate long-term treatment outcome in cervical cancer.

3D MR Volumetry for Response Assessment and Outcome Prediction

Most clinical utilization of MRI for tumor volume assessment has consisted of one- or two-dimensional diameter-based measurement using World Health Organization (WHO) (1) or Response Evaluation Criteria in Solid Tumors (RECIST) (2) principles, and most has been obtained pretherapy (24–28). Pre- and posttherapy comparisons suggest that resolution of tumor signal on the T2-weighetd MRI 3 to 6 months posttherapy is associated with better outcome (29,30). While this information is useful, it is not available until relatively late, not allowing *intratherapy* adaptation. Recent studies have shown that treatment outcome predictions can be made earlier even *within* the therapy course if higher-precision 3D tumor volumetry is employed. While WHO- and RECIST-based diameter-based measurements have difficulty accounting for complex geometric shapes, 3D measurements can accurately measure volumes with irregular geometric contours. This becomes particularly important when assessing tumor regression, because cervical cancers do not regress in a linear or concentric fashion, and become increasingly irregular in geometry during therapy (31).

Serial 3D MRI obtained at various treatment time points detects early subtle morphologic changes related to ongoing radiation/chemotherapy (Figure 1) (31), which critically influence the ultimate treatment outcome. The greater accuracy of 3D tumor volume measurements translates into an increased power for early outcome prediction. Comparisons of outcome prediction based on 3D MRI volumetry with diameter-based imaging assessments using ellipsoid computation of tumor diameters have shown that 3D MRI tumor volumetry is superior by predicting statistically

(A) MRI 1

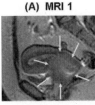

(B) MRI 2

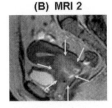

(C) MRI 3

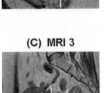

(D) MRI 4

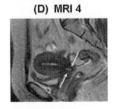

FIGURE 1 Velocity of tumor regression using serial 3D MRI in cervical cancer—rapid response, high slope, and low AUC. Serial MRI in a 41-year-old woman with a 7-cm stage IIB squamous cell carcinoma of the cervix. (A) Sagittal T2-weighted image of MRI 1 shows a well-circumscribed tumor (arrows) of the cervix. (B) MRI 2 at a cumulative dose of 19.8 Gy in 11 fractions (2 weeks) reveals tumor regression to a proportional volume of 89%. (C) In MRI 3 at 43.2 Gy in 24 fractions (5 weeks), the proportional volume is 4%. (D) The rapid response is illustrated by the regression slope of 2.2%/Gy and the AUC of 24%. The patient is alive and well 6 years and 11 months after therapy completion.

Source: Reprinted with permission from Ref. (23).

significant differences in local control rate compared with diameter-based MRI measurements (32). This predictive accuracy is likely attributable to the improved ability of the 3D MRI in delineating the tumor extent, differentiating fibrosis from tumor (9,30) and accounting for irregular configurations (31).

Based on 3D MRI volumetry, Mayr et al. (20) have studied tumor regression during the course of radiation/chemotherapy in 17 patients, and found that significant and early prediction of treatment failure can be made 4 to 5 weeks into treatment. Patients with a residual tumor volume of <20% of the pre-treatment volume at 4 to 5 weeks of therapy had a 97% local control and 72% disease-specific survival rate, compared with 53% and 50%, respectively, in patients with slower tumor regression. Similarly in a series of 42 patients, Hatano

et al. (19) found no local failures in patients with intratreatment tumor volume regression to <30% at a dose level of 30 Gy. These data suggest that serial 3D volumetry provides an indirect early assessment of the tumor's inherent responsiveness to ongoing cytotoxic therapy. In a more recent series of 115 cervical cancer patients, serial tumor regression was quantitated as regression slope and area under the regression curve (AUC). Local control increased progressively with increasingly steep slopes, to >85% with slopes of >2%/Gy, compared with <45% with slopes <1%/Gy. AUC correlated inversely with local control. Disease-specific and overall survival showed similar correlation (23).

Radiobiological response model parameters based on tumor volume regression are beginning to emerge (22,33,34). In 2006, a kinetic model to analyze MRI-based tumor regression data in cervical cancer was reported (33). Investigators at the Princess Margaret Hospital have developed a similar model based on tumor volumes from serial MRI obtained weekly during external-beam RT, and correlated model parameters with tumor hypoxia (22). These two kinetic models fit well to the temporal MRI-based 3D volume data, yielding consistent model parameters for surviving fraction (S_2) after 2 Gy and dead-cell resolving time $T_{1/2}$ (33) and T_c (22). The model parameters S_2 and $T_{1/2}$ correlated significantly with clinical outcome (34).

■ FUNCTIONAL MRI ASSESSMENT OF CERVICAL CANCER

Despite same stage and morphologic tumor volume, outcome can vary widely in cervical cancer because of different inherent biological tumor properties. The importance of functional/biological properties is well-known and related to inherent variations in vascular density and hypoxia (35,36), proliferation (36), energy metabolism, and gene expression (37,38). This variability critically influences individual patient's treatment outcome (39–42) and cannot be appreciated by the tumor's anatomic/morphologic parameter alone. Functional MRI can provide information reflecting the status of tumor perfusion, hypoxia, cellularity, and proliferation in individual patients. Its temporal changes during treatment enable early personalized prediction of ultimate treatment failure related to an ongoing treatment.

DCE MRI: Rationale and Methodology

The success of cytotoxic therapy is greatly influenced by (a) the presence and degree of hypoxic subvolumes (43–45) and (b) the effectiveness of vascular delivery of oxygen and therapeutic agents into the interstitial space within the heterogeneous tumor (46,47). The impact of hypoxia is particularly important in cervical cancer with ample evidence suggesting that hypoxia-imparted radioresistance is clinically significant (39–42,48,49). Both oxygenation and chemotherapy delivery depend on tumor perfusion, including the ability of oxygen and therapeutic agents to be delivered to the tumor region and from the vasculature into the interstitial space and to the tumor cells.

DCE MRI has been applied experimentally and clinically to characterize tumor microvascular structure and function (50–56). DCE MRI reflects tumor microcirculation, perfusion, and indirectly oxygenation status (52,57–59). Low dynamic enhancement correlates with hypxia in needle oxymetry studies (60,61) and radiobiologic hypoxic fraction in cervical cancer xenograft models (62). These translational correlates are the basis for DCE MRI's ability to provide critical information on the effective delivery of oxygen to tumor cells, which profoundly influence the therapy responsiveness, ultimate tumor control, and survival (42,63–66). Despite different imaging techniques, data analysis and tumor types, DCE MRI has shown considerable clinical relevance for prediction of outcome to cytotoxic therapy.

DCE Methods

DCE MRI consists of fast image acquisitions using T1-weighted pulse sequences before and during rapid injection of MRI contrast agents. Over a period of time, the signal intensity (SI) of the tumor, reflecting the uptake of contrast agent, can be used to create a tumor DCE SI–time curve, which can be used to characterize the tumor perfusion characteristics and derive DCE parameters.

The DCE SI–time curve has three distinct phases: upslope, plateau, and washout. Theoretical approaches have been proposed to quantify these DCE MRI parameters using multi-compartmental models (50,52,67–77). For extracranial tumors, the plateau SI and upslope of the DCE curve approximates the arterial microcirculation or tumor perfusion, based on the *first-pass* pharmacokinetic model (52,59). Our methodology for cervical cancer applied the *first-pass* DCE analysis (59) by continuously imaging the tumor dynamically before and during the arrival of the contrast bolus following fast injection of gadolinium contrast (78). This approach approximates primarily the tumor's arterial blood supply and reflects the effectiveness of the delivery of chemotherapy and oxygen. It is generally recognized that the upslope gradient in tumors is highly dependent on tissue perfusion and permeability, with perfusion predominating principally due to high blood volume and high *first-pass* extraction. The plateau SI is related to the total uptake concentration of the contrast agent in the arterial and interstitial spaces, which forms the basis for effective delivery of oxygen and chemotherapy agents, critical components for successful RT and chemotherapy, respectively.

For the *two-compartmental* analysis using a slower injection rate, the washout rate is associated with decrease of tissue contrast agent concentration (washout of the contrast) and is reported to be strongly related to vascular permeability (74,75). Although the K_{el}, or other equivalent parameters related to contrast washout, is an indirect indication of the arterial blood supply to the tumor, we prefer the *first-pass* DCE method using a fast bolus injection and analysis of the earlier arterial phase of the DCE uptake curve, which more reflects the effectiveness of chemotherapy and oxygen delivery to the tumor. In addition, the short acquisition time and rapid bolus injection shorten the MRI examination and provide higher signal-to-noise ratio for better quantitative analysis.

■ FUNCTIONAL MRI–BASED EARLY OUTCOME PREDICTION

Clinical correlations of DCE MRI with tumor control and survival have suggested that the functional assessment of tumor microcirculation provided by DCE MRI may be useful to monitor response to therapy and, more significantly, predict ultimate therapy outcome in cervical cancer. Overall, low DCE (Figure 2), signaling poor tumor perfusion and hypoxia, has been found to correlate with unfavorable treatment outcome in patients with cervical cancer (51,53,79–84).

(A1)   (B1)

Anatomical
structural
Imaging:
Tumor Delineation
T2-weighted MRI

Physiological
functional
imaging:
DCE MRI

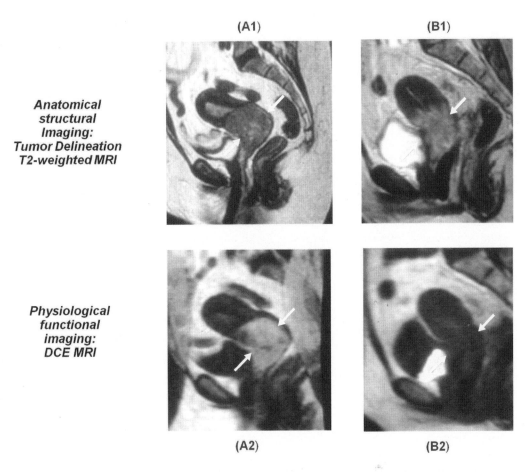

(A2)   (B2)

FIGURE 2 Anatomic/morphologic MRI and imaging and DCE MRI. Serial MRI in a 50-year-old woman with stage IIB squamous cell carcinoma of the cervix (A) and a 48-year-old woman with a stage IIB squamous cell carcinoma (B). Sagittal T2-weighted images show in the cervical tumor (arrows) in both patients (A1, B1, top). The DCE MRI of patient A shows intense enhancement in the tumor region (A2, bottom), whereas poor enhancement is observed in patient B (B2). Patient A maintained tumor control and is alive and well 7.5 years after therapy completion. Patient B developed a local recurrence 5 months after therapy and died 6 months later.

Source: Reprinted with permission from Ref. (89).

In 1996, Mayr and coworkers (51) reported the results of a pilot study investigating *first-pass* tumor perfusion pattern at pretherapy, early therapy (after a radiation dose of 20–22 Gy in 2–2.5 weeks), midtherapy (after 40–45 Gy, 4–5 weeks), and posttherapy (4–6 weeks after completion of the entire course of RT) time points. Pelvic tumor recurrence was correlated with the mean enhancement, averaged over the tumor region, in the pretherapy DCE MRI ($p = .05$), and, particularly in the MRI obtained early in the course of RT (at 20–25 Gy at 2 weeks of treatment; $p = .002$).

Yamashita et al. (85) investigated pretherapy DCE MRI in 36 cervical cancer patients. DCE was evaluated qualitatively with respect to overall intensity and homogeneity of enhancement and quantitatively by computing the capillary permeability from the SI curve. Homogenously intense enhancement correlated with better treatment response (90%) than poor or irregular ring-like enhancement (31%, $p < .1$).

In 2002, Loncaster and colleagues (79) demonstrated in 50 patients that the combination of pretherapy mean DCE MRI parameters (averaged over selected tumor regions) with tumor volume analysis correlated with outcome. The two-compartment model and plateau SI were used. Large and poorly enhanced tumors were associated with significantly worse disease-specific survival than small well-enhanced tumors (55% vs. 92%, p = .0054).

Serial DCE during Therapy and Temporal Shift of DCE

Changes in tumor perfusion and oxygenation during or after irradiation have been demonstrated experimentally (86,87). However, very few studies examined the longitudinal perfusion behavior during fractionated irradiation in cervical cancer patients.

After the initial study reporting intratreatment DCE changes observed at 20 to 25 Gy (51), Gong et al. (84) confirmed these results by studying DCE MRI in seven patients pretherapy and after the first two 2 of treatment. In the early therapy MRI, there was a statistically significant correlation of increase in mean enhancement and peak enhancement with tumor regression. Tumor enhancement did not correlate with changes in morphologic tumor volume after the first 2 weeks of RT, suggesting that microcirculation characteristics of the tumor are more sensitive than morphologic tumor volume criteria in predicting outcome. However, no long-term follow-up data was available.

Updated results in 101 patients by Yuh and others (83), using the *first-pass* DCE method, support the above results and show that low intratherapy DCE MRI, 2 weeks into the therapy course, significantly predicts unfavorable 8-year local control and survival rates (73% vs. 100%, p = .006; and 47% vs. 79%, p = .001, respectively). The 2-week intratreatment time point may be superior to the pretherapy time point—likely because the 2-week DCE MRI incorporates early therapy-specific information of responsiveness to the ongoing treatment. Such information is not available with pretreatment imaging (83).

Lyng et al. (61,88) provided histomorphologic and physiologic correlates for these clinical observations by showing a direct correlation of DCE MRI with needle-oxymetry-based tumor oxygenation, and an inverse relationship between DCE and tumor cell density in cervical cancer. In a sequential needle oxymentry and DCE MRI study, increase in oxygenation during the early RT phase was associated with a large decrease in cell density (88). These correlative findings support the hypothesis that temporal changes

in DCE during fractionated RT are indicative of changes in blood supply and tumor cell oxygenation, and may influence the efficacy of radiation-induced cell kill as reflected in the changes in intratreatment tumor cellularity (51).

These factors critically influence ultimate therapy outcome, providing the translational link between the observed imaging phenomena and clinical tumor response, local control, and survival. In a clinical outcome study of sequential DCE pretherapy, at 20 to 25 Gy, and at 45 to 50 Gy intratherapy, the impact of the temporal shift of DCE during the therapy course on local control and survival has been recently validated (Figures 3 and 4) (81). In patients with low pretherapy DCE, the sooner in the treatment course the transition from low to high DCE occurred, the more favorable were local control and survival.

Combination of Tumor Volume and Functional Parameters for Early Outcome Prediction

With tumor volume remaining a very important outcome predictor, the combination of volume and DCE parameters will be expected to improve response assessment and outcome prediction. This concept has been explored in several studies. The study by Loncaster and coworkers (79) also incorporated tumor volume measurements. Large and poorly enhanced tumors were associated with significantly worse disease-specific survival than small well-enhanced tumors (55% vs. 92%, p = .0054). Similarly a study of 16 cervical cancer patients, evaluating sequential 3D tumor volume and DCE before and during treatment, found that combination of DCE parameters with 3D volume improved response assessment and prediction of local failure in tumors with intermediate volumes of 40 to 100 cm^3 (89).

Heterogeneity Assessment of DCE

Functional tumor heterogeneity exists not only among individual patients, but also within the same tumor in each patient. However, most studies have measured the mean DCE by averaging DCE over the entire tumor volume or over partial volumes in selected regions-of-interest within the tumor (79,80,84).

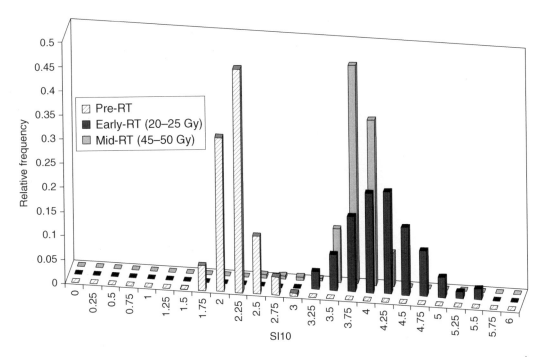

FIGURE 3 Changes in DCE pattern during the course of therapy. In this stage IB2 cervical cancer patient, the pretherapy DCE MRI revealed low DCE (cross-hatched bar, SI10 = 1.6). DCE improved in early chemoradiotherapy (dark gray bar, SI10 = 3.2) and continued to be high midway through therapy (light gray bar, SI10 = 2.7). The tumor remained locally controlled and the patient was alive and well 4 years and 10 months after therapy completion.

Source: Reprinted with permission from Ref. (81).

More recently, the concept of heterogeneity evaluation of DCE MRI has been introduced (82,83,90). A voxel-wise approach has been developed to characterize *each tumor voxel's* perfusion status to assess heterogeneity by quantifying variations of low-DCE subvolumes, indicative of poor perfusion, hypoxia and therapy-resistance, within the tumor mass (82,90).

There is ample evidence that such heterogeneous functional/biological properties within tumors correlate with treatment outcome (66,91,92) and that treatment failure is critically influenced by low-perfusion hypoxic subregions within the heterogeneous tumor (40–42,63,64,93).

In the voxel-wise analysis, the DCE voxel-histogram of SI, representing the heterogeneous distribution of DCE throughout the tumor, separates and quantitates the low-DCE voxels within the heterogeneous tumor (82,83). From the voxel histogram of SI, the concept of SI percentiles and percentile thresholds

was derived. For example, the 10th percentile of SI (SI10) <2.5 defines tumors, where the lowest 10% of tumor pixels have an SI <2.5.

Clinical correlation shows that SI10 obtained intratreatment 2 weeks into the treatment course, predicted an 88% local recurrence rate for SI10 < 2.5 versus 0% for SI10 $\geq$ 2.5 (p = .0004) (90). Further analysis of 101 patients confirmed these findings and demonstrated that the heterogeneity metric SI percentile is a better outcome predictor than the mean SI averaged over the entire tumor region (83).

■ COMBINATION OF DCE WITH OTHER MRI AND CLINICAL RESPONSE PREDICTORS

Comparison of heterogeneity DCE parameters, tumor volume, and established clinical prognosticators (stage, lymph node status, and histology) have

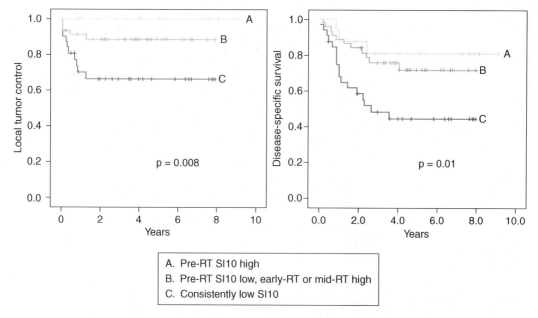

FIGURE 4 Outcome correlation of DCE changes during therapy—local control and overall survival in patients with high pretherapy DCE versus low pretherapy DCE with subsequent increase versus persistently low DCE. Kaplan–Meier curves show the three patient groups with high pretherapy DCE (Line A), consistent with initially high perfusion, low pretherapy DCE with subsequent increase in DCE (Line B), and persistently low DCE from the pretherapy throughout the midtherapy phase (Line C). Local tumor control, disease-specific survival, and overall survival are shown. The 5-year local tumor control rates are 100%, 89%, and 66%, respectively (p = .008). The 5-year disease-specific survival rates are 81%, 72%, and 44%, respectively (p = .010), and the overall survival rates are 81%, 62%, and 43%, respectively (p = .048).

Source: Reprinted with permission from Ref. (81).

shown that SI10 and residual 3D volume at 2 weeks intratherapy were significant independent and superior predictors for tumor recurrence ($p = .04$, $p = .03$) and cancer death ($p = .03$, $p < .001$) compared with the clinical prognosticators (82). Synergizing the classic prognosticators with the DCE MRI parameters, SI10 and 3D tumor, volume, increased the sensitivity and specificity of the clinical prognosticators from 71% and 51% to 100% and 71% for predicting recurrence; and from 79% and 54% to 93% and 60% for predicting death (82).

The predictive power of the DCE can also be further improved by synergizing it with hemoglobin (Hgb) levels, as a measure of the systemic oxygenation carrier capacity during therapy. In patients with both low mean Hgb levels (<11.2 g/dl) and low DCE (SI10 < 2.0) in the early treatment phase, local recurrence was significantly higher ($p = .005$) and disease-specific survival lower ($p = .056$) than in all other groups (Figure 5) (94). Conversely, both high

Hgb levels and high perfusion predicted high 5-year tumor control and survival (100% and 78%, respectively, Figure 5).

■ DIFFUSION WEIGHTED IMAGING MRI

DWI MRI assesses the microscopic Brownian motion of extracellular water molecules in tissue (95,96) thereby characterizing the water diffusion properties and reflecting indirectly the cellularity of the studied tissue (97,98). A noninvasive technique, DWI MRI does not require intravenous contrast injection and therefore is not contraindicated in cervical cancer patients with impaired renal function. Using diffusion-weighted gradient pulse sequences, water diffusibility in the soft tissue can be quantified as the apparent diffusion coefficient (ADC).

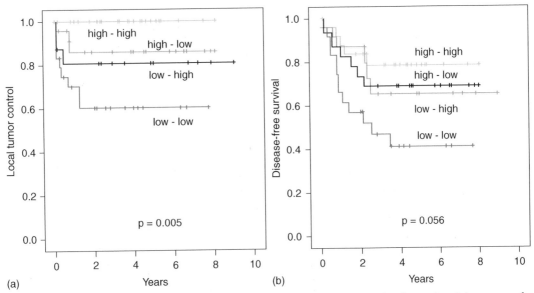

FIGURE 5 Compounded effects of DCE and mean Hgb levels during therapy on local control and disease-specific survival. Kaplan–Meier curves show tumor control (a) and disease-free survival (b) in four patient groups with high mHgb/high SI10 (high–high), high mHgb/low SI10 (high–low), low mHgb/high SI10 (low–high), and low mHgb/low SI10 (low–low) for local tumor control (a) and disease-specific survival (b). The 5-year local tumor control rates are 100%, 86%, 81%, and 60%, respectively ($p = .005$). The 5-year disease-specific survival rates are 78%, 69%, 65%, and 41%, respectively $p = .056$). The overall survival rates are 70%, 65%, 60%, and 36%, respectively ($p = .053$).

Source: Reprinted with permission from Ref. (94).

ADC is strongly influenced by the cellularity and cell membrane integrity of tumors (99). Because of restricted water motion, ADC is generally decreased in tumor tissue compared with the corresponding normal tissue (100–102). ADC values typically increase with successful treatment, when induced apoptosis and necrosis result in decreased barriers to water motion and improved water diffusibility (103,104). ADC has been recently found to be highly sensitive in quantifying subtle therapy response in gliomas (105,106), head and neck (107), and breast tumors (108). Increased ADC can be apparent within hours or days from the start of therapy, well before to before morphologic response (e.g., tumor volume change) is evident. Conversely, decrease in ADC during therapy may signal therapy resistance and treatment failure (95,105,109).

As expected, pretherapy ADC in cervical cancer is significantly lower (<1.1×10^3 mm^2/s) than in the normal cervix ($\geq 1.7 \times 10^{-3}$ mm^2/s) correlating with the higher cell density in cervical tumors compared with normal tissue (100,102). Most studies have observed an increase in mean ADC following chemoradiotherapy in patients with cervical cancer (100,110,111).

Recent early clinical experience in cervical cancer has suggested that an intratreatment increase in ADC is associated with improved tumor response after RT and chemotherapy (100,110,111). Harry et al. (110) showed in a series of 20 patients that, ADC increased significantly at 2 weeks into chemoradiotherapy, which correlated with better post-therapy tumor response. However, no longer-term follow-up data on ultimate local control and survival is available.

Similarly, Liu et al. (111) found that ADCs early in the treatment course, after 15 days of RT, increased significantly compared with pretreatment ADC ($p = .001$), while there was no statistically significant change in morphologic tumor size. The ADC values 4 weeks into therapy increased significantly over the pretreatment ADC ($p < .001$) in patients who subsequently attained a complete response. In women achieving a partial response, only small increases in ADC were observed, suggesting that persistently high cellularity during treatment is a subtle indicator of lacking therapy responsiveness.

These early studies suggest that DWI MRI shows promise as an indirect measure of tumor cellularity and as early biomarker for tumor responsiveness in cervical cancer treated with radiation/chemotherapy. Further investigations will be required to confirm that ADC parameters are correlated not only with tumor response, but also with ultimate local tumor control and disease-free survival.

■ CONCLUSIONS AND FUTURE DIRECTIONS

Anatomical/morphologic tumor volume assessment and functional MRI techniques provide imaging parameters that correlate with tumor responsiveness and treatment outcome. The high spatial resolution MRI–based tumor volumetry is advantageous over simple one- or two-diameter measurements. Functional MRI–derived imaging biomarkers, including DCE and DWI, parameters reflect the underlying pathophysiology and biological properties of the tumor and its response to an ongoing treatment, and can further enhance the ability for early prediction of ultimate treatment outcome, local control and survival. The early outcome prediction provided by these advanced imaging techniques is potentially applicable for risk-adapted therapy decision-making in cervical cancer. The predictive power can be significantly increased by augmenting morphologic 3D volumetric and functional imaging parameters with the traditional clinical prognosticators. Such an approach holds promise to provide an effective personalized and therapy-specific algorithm for early outcome prediction that may improve the ultimate therapy outcome in cervical cancer.

■ REFERENCES

1. WHO Handbook for reporting results of cancer treatment, Publication Number 48. Geneva: World Health Organization. 1979 (http://whqlibdoc.who.int.publications/9241700483.pdf).

2. James K, Eisenhauer E, Christian M, et al. Measuring response in solid tumors: Unidimensional versus bidimensional measurement. *J Natl Cancer Inst.* 1999;91:523–528.

3. Kastritis E, Bamias A, Efstathiou E, et al. The outcome of advanced or recurrent non-squamous carcinoma of the uterine cervix after platinum-based combination chemotherapy. *Gynecol Oncol.* 2005;99:376–382.

4. Chemoradiotherapy for Cervical Cancer Meta-analysis Collaboration (CCCMAC). Reducing uncertainties about the effects of chemoradiotherapy for cervical cancer: Individual patient data meta-analysis. *J Clin Oncol.* 2008;26(35):5802–5812.

5. Dueñas-González A, Zarba JJ, Alcedo JC, et al. A phase III study comparing concurrent gemcitabine (Gem) plus cisplatin (Cis) and radiation followed by adjuvant Gem plus Cis versus concurrent Cis and radiation in patients with stage IIB to IVA carcinoma of the cervix (abst). *J Clin Oncol.* 2009;27:18s.

6. Haie-Meder C, Potter R, Van Limbergen E, et al. Recommendations from Gynaecological (GYN) GEC-ESTRO Working Group (I): Concepts and terms in 3D image based 3D treatment planning in cervix cancer brachytherapy with emphasis on MRI assessment of GTV and CTV. *Radiother Oncol.* 2005;74(3):235–245.

7. Potter R, Kirisits C, Fidarova EF, et al. Present status and future of high-precision image guided adaptive brachytherapy for cervix carcinoma. *Acta Oncol.* 2008;47(7):1325–1336.

8. Hricak H, Lacey CG, Sandles LG, et al. Invasive cervical carcinoma: Comparison of MR imaging and surgical findings. *Radiology.* 1988;166:623–631.

9. Subak L, Hricak H, Powell CB, et al. Cervical carcinoma: Computed tomography and magnetic resonance imaging for preoperative staging. *Obstet Gynecol.* 1995;86(1):43–50.

10. Mitchell D, Snyder B, Coakley F, et al. Early invasive cervical cancer: Tumor delineation by magnetic resonance imaging, computed tomography, and clinical examination, verified by pathologic results, in the ACRIN 6651/GOG 183 Intergroup Study. *J Clin Oncol.* 2006;24:5687–5694.

11. Burghardt E, Hofmann HM, Ebner F, et al. Magnetic resonance imaging in cervical cancer: A basis for objective classification. *Gynecol Oncol.* 1989;33:61–67.

12. Greco A, Mason P, Leung AWL, et al. Staging of carcinoma of the uterine cervix: MR-surgical correlation. *Clin Radiol.* 1989;40:401–405.

13. Rubens D, Thornbury JR, Angel C, et al. Stage IB cervical carcinoma: Comparison of clinical, MR, and pathologic staging. *AJR.* 1988;150:135–138.

14. Kim SH, Choi BI, Lee HP, et al. Uterine cervical carcinoma: Comparison of CT and MR findings. *Radiology.* 1990;175:45–51.

15. Eifel PJ, Morris M, Wharton JT, et al. The influence of tumor size and morphology on the outcome of patients with FIGO stage IB squamous cell carcinoma of the uterine cervix. *Int J Radiat Oncol Biol Phys.* 1994;29:9–16.

16. Kovalic JJ, Perez CA, Grigsby PW, et al. The effect of volume of disease in patients with carcinoma of the uterine cervix. *Int J Radiat Oncol Biol Phys.* 1991;21:905–910.

17. Lowrey GC, Mendenhall MW, Million RR. Stage IB or IIA-B carcinoma of the intact uterine cervix treated with irradiation: A multivariate analysis. *Int J Radiat Oncol Biol Phys.* 1992;24:205–210.

18. Perez CA, Grigsby P, Nene S, et al. Effect of tumor size on the prognosis of carcinoma of the uterine cervix treated with irradiation alone. *Cancer.* 1992;69:2796–2806.

19. Hatano K, Sekiya Y, Araki H, et al. Evaluation of the therapeutic effect of radiotherapy on cervical cancer using magnetic resonance imaging. *Int J Radiat Oncol Biol Phys.* 1999;45:693–644.

20. Mayr NA, Magnotta VA, Ehrhardt JC, et al. Usefulness of tumor volumetry by magnetic resonance imaging in assessing response to radiation therapy in carcinoma of the uterine cervix. *Int J Radiat Oncol Biol Phys.* 1996;35(5):915–924.

21. Sethi TK, Bhalla NK, Jena AN, et al. Magnetic resonance imaging in carcinoma cervix—does it have a prognostic relevance. *J Cancer Res Ther.* 2005;1(2):103–107.

22. Lim K, Chan P, Dinniwell R, Fyles A, et al. Cervical cancer regression measured using weekly magnetic resonance imaging during fractionated radiotherapy: Radiobiologic modeling and correlation with tumor hypoxia. *Int J Radiat Oncol Biol Phys.* 2008;70(1):126–133.

23. Mayr NA, Wang JZ, Lo SS, et al. Translating response during therapy into ultimate treatment outcome: A personalized 4-Dimensional MRI tumor volumetric regression approach in cervical cancer. *Int J Radiat Oncol Biol Phys.* 2010;76(3):719–727.

24. Kim H, Kim W, Lee M, et al. Tumor volume and uterine body invasion assessed by MRI for prediction of outcome in cervical carcinoma treated with concurrent chemotherapy and radiotherapy. *Jpn J Clin Oncol.* 2007;37(11):858–866.

25. Kodaira T, Fuwa N, Kamata M, et al. Clinical assessment by MRI for patients with stage II cervical carcinoma treated by radiation alone in multicenter analysis: Are all patients with stage II disease suitable candidates for chemo-therapy? *Int J Rad Oncol Biol Phys.* 2002;52(3):627–636.

26. Wagenaar HC, Trimbos JB, Postema S, Anastasopoulou A, et al. Tumor diameter and volume assessed by magnetic resonance imaging in the prediction of outcome for invasive cervical cancer. *Gynecol Oncol.* 2001;82:474–482.

27. Hricak H, Powell CB, Yu KK, et al. Invasive cervical carcinoma: Role of MR imaging in pretreatment workup—cost-minimization and diagnosis efficacy. *Radiology.* 1996;198:403–409.

28. Hricak H, Quivey J, Campos Z, et al. Carcinoma of the cervix: Predictive value of clinical and magnetic resonance (MR) imaging assessment of prognostic factors. *Int J Radiat Oncol Biol Phys.* 1993;27:791–801.

29. Flueckiger F, Ebner F, Poschauko H, et al. Cervical cancer: Serial MR imaging before and after primary radiation therapy—a 2-year follow-up study. *Radiology.* 1992;184:89–93.

30. Hricak H. Cancer of the uterus: The value of MRI pre-and post-irradiation. *Int J Rad Oncol Biol Phys.* 1991;21:1089–1094.

31. Mayr NA, Yuh WTC, Taoka T, et al. Serial therapy-induced changes in tumor shape in cervical cancer and their impact on assessing tumor volume and treatment response. *AJR Am J Roentgenol.* 2006;187:65–72.

32. Mayr NA, Taoka T, Yuh WT, et al. Method and timing of tumor volume measurement for outcome prediction in cervical cancer using magnetic resonance imaging. *Int J Radiat Oncol Biol Phys.* 2002;52(1):14–22.

33. Wang JZ, Mayr NA, Yuh WTC, et al. Kinetic Model of Tumor Regression During Radiation Therapy of Cervical Cancer (abstr). *Int J Radiat Oncol Biol Phys.* 2006;66:603.

34. Huang Z, Mayr NA, Yuh WTC, et al. Predicting outcomes in cervical cancer: A kinetic model of tumor regression during radiation therapy. *Cancer Res.* 2010;70(2):463–470.

35. Delorme S, Knopp MV. Non-invasive vascular imaging: Assessing tumour vascularity [Review]. *European Radiology.* 1998;8(4):517–527.

36. Pugachev A, Ruan S, Carlin S. Dependence of FDG uptake on tumor microenvironment. *Int J Radiat Oncol Biol Phys.* 2005;62:545–553.

37. Bachtiary B, Boutros PC, Pintilie M. Gene expression profiling in cervical cancer: An exploration of intratumor heterogeneity. *Clin Cancer Res.* 2006;12:5632–5640.

38. Zhao S, Kuge Y, Mochizuki T. Biologic correlates of intratumoral heterogeneity in 18F-FDG distribution with regional expression of glucose transporters and hexokinase-II in experimental tumor. *J Nucl Med.* 2005;46:675–682.

39. Hockel M, Schlenger K, Aral B, et al. Association between tumor hypoxia and malignant progression in advanced cancer of the uterine cervix. *Cancer Res.* 1996;56:4509–4515.

40. Bush RS, Jenkin RDT, Allt WEC. Definitive evidence for hypoxic cells influencing cure in cancer therapy. *Br J Cancer.* 1978;37(Suppl 3):302–306.

41. Kolstad P. Intercapillary distance, oxygen tension and local recurrence in cervix cancer. *Scand J Clin Lab Invest.* 1968;106(Suppl):145–157.

42. Vaupel P. Oxygenation of solid tumors. In: Teicher BA, eds. *Drug Resistance in Oncology.* Marcel Dekker, Inc. New York. 1993:53–85.

43. Gray LH, Conger AD, Ebert M. The concentration of oxygen dissolved in tissues at the time of irradiation as a factor in radiotherapy. *Br J Radiol.* 1953;26:638–648.

44. Trotter MJ, Chaplin DJ, Durand RE, et al. The use of fluorescent probes to identify regions of transient

perfusion in murine tumors. *Int J Rad Oncol Biol Phys.* 1989;16:931–934.

45. Overgaard J, Horsman MR. Modification of hypoxia-induced radio-resistance in tumors by the use of oxygen and sensitizers. *Semin Radiat Oncol.* 1996;6:10–21.

46. Meta-analysis Group in Cancer. Efficacy of intravenous continuous infusion of fluorouracil compared with bolus administration in advanced colorectal cancer (abst). *J Clin Oncol.* 1998;16:301–308.

47. Link KH, Leder G, Pillasch J. In vitro concentration response studies and in vitro phase II tests as the experimental basis for regional chemotherapeutic protocols. *Semin Surg Oncol.* 1998;14:189–201.

48. Mendenhall WM, Thar TL, Bova FJ, et al. Prognostic and treatment factors affecting pelvic control of stage IB and IIA-B carcinoma of the intact uterine cervix treated with radiation therapy alone. *Cancer.* 1984;53:2649–2654.

49. Thomas G. The effect of hemoglobin level on radiotherapy outcomes: The Canadian experience. *Semin Oncol.* 2001;28 (S8):60–65.

50. Brix G, Rempp K, Guckel F. Quantitative assessment of tissue microcirculation by dynamic contrast-enhanced MR imaging. *Adv MRI Contrast.* 1994;2:68–77.

51. Mayr NA, Yuh WTC, Magnotta VA, et al. Tumor perfusion studies using fast magnetic resonance imaging technique in advanced cervical cancer—a new noninvasive predictive assay. *Int J Radiat Oncol Biol Phys.* 1996;36:623–633.

52. Tofts PS, Brix G, Buckley DL, et al. Estimating kinetic parameters from dynamic contrast-enhanced T1-weighted MRI of a diffusable tracer: Standardized quantities and symbols. *J Magn Reson.* 1999;10:223–232.

53. Hawighorst H, Knapstein PG, Knopp MV, et al. Uterine cervical carcinoma: Comparison of standard and pharmacokinetic analysis of time-intensity curves for assessment of tumor angiogenesis and patient survival. *Cancer Res.* 1998;58:3598–3602.

54. Hoskins PJ, Saunders MI, Goodchild K, et al. Dynamic contrast enhanced magnetic resonance scanning as a predictor of response to accelerated radiotherapy for advanced head and neck cancer. *Br J Radiol.* 1999;72: 1093–1098.

55. Koukourakis MI, Giatromanolaki A, Sivridis E, et al. Cancer vascularization: Implications in radiotherapy? *Int J Rad Oncol Biol Phys.* 2000;48:545–553.

56. Reddick WE, Taylor JS, Fletcher BD. Dynamic MR imaging (DEMRI) of microcirculation in bone sarcoma. *J Magn Reson Imaging.* 1999;10:277–285.

57. Evelhoch JL. Key factors in the acquisition of contrast kinetic data for oncology. *J Magn Reson Imaging.* 1999;10:254–259.

58. Taylor JS, Tofts PS, Port RE, et al. MR imaging of tumor microcirculation: Promise for the new millennium. *J Magn Reson Imaging.* 1999;10:903–907.

59. Yuh WTC. An exciting and challenging role for the advanced contrast MR imaging. *J Magn Reson Imaging.* 1999;10:221–222.

60. Cooper RA, Carrington BM, Loncaster JA, et al. Tumour oxygenation levels correlate with dynamic contrast-enhanced magnetic resonance imaging parameters in carcinoma of the cervix. *Radiother Oncol.* 2000;57:53–59.

61. Lyng H, Vorren AO, Sundfør K, et al. Assessment of tumor oxygenation in human cervical carcinoma by use of dynamic Gd-DTPA-enhanced MR imaging. *J Magn Reson Imaging.* 2001;14:750–756.

62. Ellingsen C, Natvig I, Gaustad JV, et al. Human cervical carcinoma xenograft models for studies of the physiological microenvironment of tumors. *J Cancer Res Clin Oncol.* 2009;135(9):1177–1184.

63. Höckel M, Schlenger K, Mitze M, et al. Hypoxia and radiation response in human tumors. *Semin Radiat Oncol.* 1996;6:3–9.

64. Dunst J, Kuhnt T, Strauss HG, et al. Anemia in cervical cancers: Impact on survival, patterns of relapse, and association with hypoxia and angiogenesis. *Int J Radiat Oncol Biol Phys.* Jul 2003;56(3):778–787.

65. Minchinton AI, Tannock IF. Drug penetration in solid tumours. *Nat Rev Cancer.* Aug 2006;6(8):583–592.

66. Galmarini FC, Galmarini CM, Sarchi MI, et al. Heterogeneous distribution of tumor blood supply affects the response to chemotherapy in patients with head and neck cancer. *Microcirculation.* 2000;7:405–410.

67. Brix G, Semmler W, Port R, Schad LR, et al. Pharmacokinetic parameters in CNS Gd-DTPA enhanced MR imaging. *J Comput Assist Tomogr.* 1991;15:621–727.

68. Brix G, Schreiber W, Hoffmann U, et al. Methodological approaches to quantitative evaluation of microcirculation in tissues with dynamic magnetic resonance tomography [Review]. *Radiologe.* 1997;37(6):470–480.

69. Daniel BL, Yen YF, Glover GH, et al. Breast disease: Dynamic spiral MR imaging. *Radiology.* 1998;209: 499–509.

70. Griebel J, Mayr NA, deVries A, et al. Assessment of tumor microcirculation—a new role of dynamic contrast MR imaging. *J Magn Reson Imaging.* 1997;7:111–119.

71. Kety S. The theory and application of the exchange of inert gas at the lungs and tissues. *Pharmacol Rev.* 1951;3: 1–41.

72. Kuhl CK, Mielcareck P, Klaschik S, et al. Dynamic breast MR imaging: Are signal intensity time course data useful for differential diagnosis of enhancing lesions? *Radiology.* 1999;211:101–110.

73. Larsson H, Stubgaard M, Frederiksen L, et al. Quantitation of blood-brain barrier defect by magnetic resonance imaging and Gadolinium-DTPA in patients with multiple sclerosis and brain tumors. *Magn Reson Med.* 1990;16:117–131.

74. Su MY, Jao J, Nalcioglu O. Measurement of vascular volume fraction and blood-tissue permeability constants with a pharmacokinetic model: Studies in rat muscle tumors with dynamic Gd-DTPA enhanced MRI. *Magn Reson Med.* 1994;32:714–724.

75. Su MY, Cheung YC, Fruehauf JP, et al. Correlation of dynamic contrast enhancement MRI parameters with microvessel density and VEGF for assessment of angiogenesis in breast cancer. *J Magn Reson Imaging.* 2003;18:467–477.

76. Tofts PS, Kermode AG. Measurement of the blood-brain barrier permeability and leakage space using dynamic MR imaging: Fundamental concepts. *Magn Reson Med.* 1991;17:357–367.

77. Tofts PS. Modeling tracer kinetics in dynamic Gd-DTPA MR imaging. *J Magn Reson Imaging.* 1997;7:91–101.

78. Daldrup HE, Shames DM, Husseini W, et al. Quantification of the extraction fraction for gadopentetate across breast cancer capillaries. *Magn Reson Med.* 1998;40:537–543.

79. Loncaster JA, Carrington BM, Sykes JR, et al. Prediction of radiotherapy outcome using dynamic contrast enhanced MRI of carcinoma of the cervix. *Int J Rad Oncol Biol Phys.* 2002;54:759–767.

80. Yamashita Y, Baba T, Baba Y, et al. Dynamic contrast-enhanced MR imaging of uterine cervical cancer: Pharmacokinetic analysis with histopathologic correlation and its importance in predicting the outcome of radiation therapy. *Radiology.* 2000;216:803–809.

81. Mayr NA, Wang JZ, Zhang D, et al. Longitudinal changes in tumor perfusion pattern during the radiation therapy course and its clinical impact in cervical cancer. *Int J Radiat Oncol Biol Phys.* 2010;77:502–508.

82. Mayr NA, Yuh WTC, Jajoura D, et al. Ultra-early predictive assay for treatment failure using functional magnetic resonance imaging and clinical prognostic parameters in cervical cancer. *Cancer.* 2010;116(3):903–912.

83. Yuh WTC, Mayr NA, Jarjoura D, et al. Predicting control of primary tumor and survival by DCE MRI during early therapy in cervical cancer. *Invest Radiol.* 2009;44:343–350.

84. Gong QY, Brunt JN, Romaniuk CS, et al. Contrast enhanced dynamic MRI of cervical carcinoma during radiotherapy: Early prediction of tumour regression rate. *Br J Radiol.* 1999;72:1177–1184.

85. Yamashita H, Nakagawa K, Tago M, et al. Treatment results and prognostic analysis of radical radiotherapy for locally advanced cancer of the uterine cervix. *Br J Radiol.* 2005;78(933):821–826.

86. Goda F, O'Hara JA, Rhodes ES, et al. Changes of oxygen tension in experimental tumors after a single dose of X-ray irradiation. *Cancer Res.* 1995;55(11):2249–2252.

87. Yu H, Su MY, Wang Z, Nalcioglu O. A longitudinal study of radiation-induced changes in tumor vasculature by contrast-enhanced magnetic resonance imaging. *Radiat Res.* Aug 2002;2:152–158.

88. Lyng H, Sundfor K, Rofstad EK. Changes in tumor oxygen tension during radiotherapy of uterine cervical cancer: Relationships to changes in vascular density, cell density, and frequency of mitosis and apoptosis. *Int J Rad Oncol Biol Phys.* 2000;46:935–946.

89. Mayr NA, Yuh WT, Zheng J, et al. Prediction of tumor control in patients with cervical cancer: Analysis of combined volume and dynamic enhancement pattern by MR imaging. *Am J Roentgenol.* 1998;170(1):177–182.

90. Mayr NA, Yuh WTC, Arnholt JC, et al. Pixel analysis of MR perfusion imaging in predicting radiation therapy outcome in cervical cancer. *J Magn Reson Imaging.* 2000;12:1027–1033.

91. Britten RA, Evans AJ, Allalunis-Turner MJ, et al. Intratumoral heterogeneity as a confounding factor in clonogenic assays for tumour radioresponsiveness. *Radiother Oncol.* 1996;39(2):145–153.

92. Lyng H, Vorren AO, Sundfor K, et al. Intra- and inter-tumor heterogeneity in blood perfusion of human cervical cancer before treatment and after radiotherapy. *Int J Cancer.* 2001;96:182–190.

93. Weidner N. Tumoral vascularity as a prognostic factor in cancer patients: The evidence continues to grow. *J Pathol.* 1998;184:119–122.

94. Mayr A, Wang JZ, Zhang D, et al. Synergistic effects of hemoglobin and tumor perfusion on tumor control and survival in cervical cancer. *Int J Radiat Oncol Biol Phys.* 2009;74(5):1513–1521.

95. Charles-Edwards EM, deSouza NM, Diffusion-weighted magnetic resonance imaging and its application to cancer. *Cancer Imaging.* 2006;6:135–143.

96. Rowley HA, Grant PE, Roberts TP. Diffusion MR imaging: Theory and applications. *Neuroimaging Clin N Am.* 1999;9:343–361.

97. Hamstra DA, Rehemtulla A, Ross BD. Diffusion magnetic resonance imaging: A biomarker for treatment response in oncology. *J Clin Oncol.* 2007;25:4104–4109.

98. Ross BD, Moffat BA, Lawrence TS, Mukherji SK, et al. Evaluation of cancer therapy using diffusion magnetic resonance imaging. *Mol Cancer Ther.* 2003;2(6):581–587.

99. Sugahara T, Korogi Y, Kochi M, Ikushima I, et al. Usefulness of diffusion-weighted MRI with echo-planar technique in the evaluation of cellularity in gliomas. *J Magn Reson Imaging.* 1999;9(1):53–60.

100. Naganawa S, Sato C, Kumada H, Ishigaki T, et al. Apparent diffusion coefficient in cervical cancer of the uterus: Comparison with the normal uterine cervix. *Eur Radiol.* 2005;15:71–78.

101. McVeigh PZ, Syed AM, Milosevic M, et al. Diffusion-weighted MRI in cervical cancer. *Eur Radiol.* 2008;18:1058–1064.

102. Ho KC, Lin G, Wang JJ, Lai CH, et al. Correlation of apparent diffusion coefficients measured by 3T diffusion-weighted MRI and SUV from FDG PET/CT in primary cervical cancer. *Eur J Nucl Med Mol Imaging.* 2009;36:200–208.

103. Zhao M, Pipe JG, Bonnett J, Evelhoch JL. Early detection of treatment response by diffusion-weighted 1H-NMR spectroscopy in a murine tumour in vivo. *Br J Cancer.* 1996;73(1):61–64.

104. Galons JP, Altbach MI, Paine-Murrieta GD, Taylor CW, Gillies RJ. Early increases in breast tumor xenograft water mobility in response to paclitaxel therapy detected by non-invasive diffusion magnetic resonance imaging. *Neoplasia.* 1999;1(2):113–117.

105. Chenevert TL, Stegman LD, Taylor JM, Robertson PL, et al. Diffusion magnetic resonance imaging: An early surrogate marker of therapeutic efficacy in brain tumors. *J Natl Cancer Inst.* 2000;92(24):2029–2036.

106. Galbán CJ, Chenevert TL, Meyer CR, Tsien C, et al. The parametric response map is an imaging biomarker for early cancer treatment outcome. *Nat Med.* 2009;15(5):572–576.

107. Hamstra DA, Lee KC, Moffat BA, Chenevert TL, et al. Diffusion magnetic resonance imaging: An imaging treatment response biomarker to chemoradiotherapy in a mouse model of squamous cell cancer of the head and neck. *Transl Oncol.* 2008;1(4):187–194.

108. Pickles MD, Gibbs P, Lowry M, Turnbull LW. Diffusion changes precede size reduction in neoadjuvant treatment of breast cancer. *Magn Reson Imaging.* 2006;24(7):843–847.

109. Charles-Edwards EM, Messiou C, Morgan VA, De Silva SS, et al. Diffusion-weighted imaging in cervical cancer with an endovaginal technique: Potential value for improving tumor detection in stage Ia and Ib1 disease. *Radiology.* 2008;249(2):541–550.

110. Harry VN, Semple SI, Gilbert FJ, Parkin DE. Diffusion-weighted magnetic resonance imaging in the early detection of response to chemoradiation in cervical cancer. *Gynecol Oncol.* 2008;111:213–220.

111. Liu Y, Bai R, Sun H, Liu H, et al. Diffusion-weighted imaging in predicting and monitoring the response of uterine cervical cancer to combined chemoradiation. *Clin Radiol.* 2009;64:1067–1074.

Index

Note: Page numbers followed by "f" and "t" denote figures and tables, respectively.